DATE DUE		
MAR 14 1988		
MAR 21 1988		
DEC 03 1998		
1 4 MAR 2001		
April 26/02		

HEALTH EFFECTS OF
LOW-LEVEL
RADIATION

HEALTH EFFECTS OF
LOW-LEVEL
RADIATION

Editor

William R. Hendee, Ph.D.

Professor and Chairman
Department of Radiology
University of Colorado
Health Sciences Center
Denver, Colorado

APPLETON-CENTURY-CROFTS/Norwalk, Connecticut

Copyright © 1984 by Appleton-Century-Crofts
A Publishing Division of Prentice-Hall, Inc.

84 85 86 87 88 89 / 10 9 8 7 6 5 4 3 2 1

Prentice-Hall International, Inc., London
Prentice-Hall of Australia, Pty. Ltd., Sydney
Prentice-Hall of Canada, Inc.
Prentice-Hall of India Private Limited, New Delhi
Prentice-Hall of Japan, Inc., Tokyo
Prentice-Hall of Southeast Asia (Pte.) Ltd., Singapore
Whitehall Books Ltd., Wellington, New Zealand
Editora Prentice-Hall do Brasil Ltda., Rio de Janeiro

Library of Congress Cataloging in Publication Data
Main entry under title:

Health effects of low level radiation.

Bibliography: p.
Includes index.
1. Ionizing radiation — Toxicology.   2. Ionizing
radiation — Physiological effect.   I. Hendee, William R.,
1938-   . [DNLM: 1. Radiation Effects.   2. Radiation,
Ionizing — Adverse effects.   WN 620 H434]
RA1231.R2H36 1983   616.9'897   83-2708
ISBN 0-8385-3666-2

Cover and text design: Lynn Luchetti
Production: Carol Pierce

iv

Contributors

Max L. Baker, Ph.D.
Associate Professor
Department of Radiology
Chief, Division of Radiological Sciences
University of Arkansas for Medical Sciences
Little Rock, Arkansas

Glenn V. Dalrymple, M.D.
Clinical Professor of Radiology and Biometry
University of Arkansas for Medical Sciences
Little Rock, Arkansas

Marc Edwards, Ph.D.
Chief of Radiological Sciences
Department of Radiology
University of Missouri-Columbia
School of Medicine
Columbia, Missouri

Gerald P. Hanson, Ph.D.
Radiation Advisor
Division of Disease Prevention and Control
Pan American Health Organization
Washington, D.C.

William R. Hendee, Ph.D.
Professor and Chairman
Department of Radiology
University of Colorado Health Sciences Center
Denver, Colorado

Donald B. Hess, M.S.
Department of Radiology
University of Colorado Medical School
Denver, Colorado

John C. Holder, M.D.
Department of Radiology
University of Arkansas for Medical Sciences
Little Rock, Arkansas

Marilyn M. Pesto-Edwards, R.N., M.S.N., J.D.
Assistant Director, Risk Management
Missouri Professional Liability Insurance Association
Jefferson City, Missouri

Kedar N. Prasad, Ph.D.
Professor, Department of Radiology
University of Colorado Health Sciences Center
Denver, Colorado

E. Russell Ritenour, Ph.D.
Instructor, Department of Radiology
University of Colorado Health Sciences Center
Denver, Colorado

Arthur Robinson, M.D.
Professor, Department of Biochemistry and Biophysics and Genetics
University of Colorado Health Sciences Center and National Jewish
    Hospital and Research Center
Denver, Colorado

David A. Savitz, Ph.D.
Assistant Professor
Department of Preventive Medicine
University of Colorado Health Sciences Center
Denver, Colorado

Jeffrey V. Sutherland, Ph.D.
Assistant Professor
Department of Radiology
University of Colorado Health Sciences Center
Denver, Colorado

Steven R. Wilkins, Ph.D.
Instructor
Department of Radiology
University of Colorado Health Sciences Center
Denver, Colorado

Contents

Preface

Almost no topic is discussed more and understood less than that of the health effects of exposure to low levels of ionizing radiation. Any trivial incident in a nuclear power plant, whether foreseen or not, receives coverage in the national, even international, press. The disposal of small quantities of radioactive waste from research facilities and medical institutions is presented to the public as an unsolvable problem of immense proportion. Public rallys link the use of radioactivity and nuclear energy to escalation of the deployment of nuclear missiles and to an increased potential for terrorism and sabotage involving nuclear weapons. The use of radiation in medicine is described as inducing more disease than it is capable of detecting and curing.

Why is radiation identified in so emotional a fashion? Probably there are many causes. None of the physical senses is sensitive to the presence of radiation, consequently, radiation creates a state of dependency where the individual is forced to rely upon technology and the advice of scientists and technicians for his protection. Many of radiation's most vociferous opponents have been reared in an era of class B movies and television programs that present radiation and nuclear energy as the ultimate uncontrollable force capable of laying waste to vast areas of the environment and to countless human lives. For individuals needing a public forum for the topic of radiation and its philosophical expression, "hazards" is almost guaranteed to provide it.

Like most products of a modern society, radiation has both positive and negative features. The task of society is to take advantage of the positive features while minimizing the risk of the negative features. The degree to which radiation can be used to benefit mankind requires thoughtful judgment and a careful balance of protection versus cost and benefit versus risk. The judgment and balance can be arrived at only by a well-informed and unbiased public that can sift through the emotional rhetoric on both sides of the radiation issues to arrive at intelligent and useful decisions. To achieve these objectives, the public needs access to information and to individuals that present information about radiation and nuclear energy in as factual a manner as possible. The presentation of such information is the reason for this text.

Authors of the text were selected for their scientific and medical knowledge and for their unbiased approach to radiation, its beneficial uses and its health effects. Contributions of these authors provide a comprehensive overview of the topics of radiation and its health effects, and serve as an introduction to the subjects for individuals wishing to expand their knowledge about radiation and nuclear energy. Readers of the text are encouraged to seek this expanded knowledge by pursuing the references listed at the end of each chapter.

William R. Hendee
Denver, Colorado

HEALTH EFFECTS OF
LOW-LEVEL
RADIATION

1.

What Is Radiation and How Is It Produced?

Marc Edwards

The general public is exposed continuously to low-level radiation. This fact is well known to the general public, which is also exposed continuously to information and misinformation about low-level radiation and its effects on the health and well-being of the individual. Radiation exposure is present from conception; media "exposure" begins shortly thereafter. The continuing debate over nuclear energy and the more recent concerns about nuclear warfare ensure that radiation and its effects will continue to be much discussed. In fact, the point has been reached that the general public should and must have considerable knowledge about low-level radiation in order to make rational decisions concerning the conduct of peoples' personal lives, as well as the conduct of public policy.

Anyone setting out to become informed about radiation and its effects would probably be struck by the large amount of new terminology to be digested. Although the obvious starting point for this discussion is a concise definition of radiation, it is interesting to examine first the history of the word. Even though it sometimes seems that radiation is a modern phenomenon, the first English use of the word occurred in 1570 in a mathematical treatise on optics, wherein the author noted "Perspective . . . demonstrateth the manner and properties of all Radiations, Direct, Broken, and Reflected."[1] The Latin root word *radiare*, meaning "to emit rays," predates this first English usage considerably. The early concept of radiation evolved entirely around visible light, such that by 1773, the third edition of the *Encyclopedia Britannica* defined radiation as "the act of a body emitting or diffusing rays of light all round, as from a centre."[1]

One century later, it was discovered that both heat and radiowaves obeyed the same physical laws as visible light, and hence constituted "radiation" as well. By 1866, James Clerk Maxwell explained on a theoretical basis all that was then known about radiation in terms of the interaction among electric charges, electric fields, and magnetic fields. He combined the many different types of radiation into a generic class termed "electromagnetic" radiation. Although his theory was correct, experimenters soon discovered new "rays" that did not fit into his scheme.

In the late 1890s workers investigating the newly discovered phenomenon of radioactivity discovered alpha, beta, and gamma rays, while experimenters examining the behavior of electrons in vacuum tubes discovered x-rays. Some years later, cosmic rays were also discovered. The designations of α-, β-, γ-, x-, and cosmic rays were temporary symbolic assignments until their precise nature and source could be determined. Thus, x-rays were soon determined to be electromagnetic radiation, while α- and β-rays were determined to be energetic helium nuclei and electrons, respectively. Cosmic rays turned out to encompass a variety of particles ultimately arising from interactions of very high-energy protons and helium ions with the earth's atmosphere. Fortunately, physicists dropped their penchant for designating a new ray every time a new particle was discovered; otherwise, we would have even more names to deal with.

The word radiation thus came to encompass a wide range of seemingly disparate physical phenomena ranging from radiowaves to π-mesons. The common denominator in the menagerie is that all radiations are a form of energy. Hence, a current definition of radiation is "the process in which energy is emitted as particles or waves."[2]

To illustrate this rather broad definition, one may perform a "thought experiment" by defining an imaginary cube of air of dimension 1m on a side. What radiation might be discovered inside this cube? To make these "discoveries," we shall have to make use of some means of sensing or detecting the radiation. Beginning with some readily available detectors, our eyes, and a thermometer, we can immediately detect the presence of visible and thermal electromagnetic radiation. The presence of any ultraviolet electromagnetic radiation could eventually be detected by observing skin pigment changes such as tanning. The presence of radiowave electromagnetic radiation could be detected by listening to a portable AM–FM radio receiver placed in the center of the cube. Of course, most of this radiation does not originate inside the cube, but rather is just "passing through" and could be easily excluded from the cube by surrounding it with a thin metal shield. What then might be detected at the center of this "shielded" cube, and what sort of detector should be used?

To make a long story short, imagine a gold leaf electroscope, or alternatively a charged capacitor, at the center of the shielded cube. Both devices consist of positive and negative electrical charges insulated by a medium. The electroscope has the advantage of being a self-read device, whereas a voltmeter is required to assess the amount of charge on the capacitor. Assuming a perfect insulator between the opposite charges, the detectors would be expected to remain charged indefinitely. However, it is easily ascertained that both devices slowly lose their charge when positioned at the center of the shielded cube.

A few further experiments would reveal that the cause of this charge leakage is the production of positive and negative charge carriers in the insulating medium (in the present case, the insulating medium is air). These charge carriers are called ions, and the process by which they are produced is called ionization. Thus, some form of energy has been detected that is either able to penetrate the metal shield or originates from a source inside the shield and that has the ability to cause ionization.

Further experimentation as to the nature of the ionizing radiation would reveal that it originates from sources both outside and inside the shielded cube. The external sources are attributable to penetrating radiations from the interaction of primary cosmic rays in the atmosphere, as well as for penetrating radiation from the decay of radioactive isotopes in the environment. The internal sources are attributable to gaseous radioactive isotopes in the air, primarily radon. Of all the types of electromagnetic and particulate radiation, our attention will be focused on those that cause ionization, because this process is an essential step in the production of biologic damage. This is, of course, not to imply that nonionizing radiations, such as microwaves or sunlight, are harmless.

Ionizing radiation is thus seen to be energy emitted or produced as particles or waves and that, when it interacts with matter, produces negative and positive ions. Within this broad definition we may further classify ionizing radiation as to type, ionization density, and origin. The reference to "waves" is often meant to imply electromagnetic radiation, while "particle" often refers to matter with a nonzero rest mass. As previously mentioned electromagnetic radiation consists of a self-propagating combination of an electric field and a magnetic field.

Regardless of its energy, electromagnetic radiation always travels at the speed of light. The only distinguishing characteristics between types of electromagnetic radiation are wavelength and frequency. It is often convenient, particularly when describing the interaction of electromagnetic energy with matter, to use particlelike descriptors, in which case electromagnetic radiation is referred to as "photons." Both x-rays and γ-rays are ionizing electromagnetic radiation, and both are photons. The difference in terminology reflects different methods of production: x-rays are produced outside the nucleus, whereas γ-rays are produced within the nucleus.

Particulate radiation consists of elementary atomic, nuclear, and subnuclear particles that, unlike electromagnetic radiation, have a nonzero rest mass. Particulate radiation may possess either a positive or negative electric charge, or be neutral (uncharged). Given sufficient energy, all charged particulate radiation is ionizing, and most uncharged particulate radiation interacts to form ionizing secondary charged particles. For this reason, charged radiation is often called directly ionizing radiation, while uncharged radiation is called indirectly ionizing. Some commonly encountered charged particulate radiations are electrons and positrons (also termed β particles when they result from radioactive decay), α particles (helium nuclei resulting from radioactive decay), protons (often produced by neutron interactions), and various muons and pions (resulting from primary cosmic ray interactions in the atmosphere).

The most common uncharged particulate radiation is the neutron, which may be produced in nuclear fission and by a number of nuclear reactions. Although a great many more particulate radiations exist, they are produced only at very high energies, have very short lifetimes, and hence are usually not of concern, except around high-energy accelerators used in physics research.

Another method of classifying different types of radiation is by their resulting ionization density. Some radiations produce sparse ionization as they travel through and interact with matter, while others result in dense ionization. This pattern and density of ionization has very important consequences in the production of biologic damage. Rather than sparsely or densely ionizing, the terminology low-linear energy transfer (LET) and high-LET could also be used, where LET is the rate at which energy (and hence ionization) is deposited per unit distance traveled by the radiation. Some examples of sparsely ionizing, low-LET radiations are photons and electrons, while neutrons and α particles are examples of densely ionizing, high-LET radiations.

As was discovered in tracking down the site of origin of radiation in the imaginary cubic meter of air, radiation can originate either externally or internally with respect to a given volume. This classification of external versus internal radiation is often used when some particular organism, be it a cell, a mouse, or a man, is the volume of interest. Internal radiation is that radiation, both electromagnetic and particulate, that arises from sources absorbed, ingested, or somehow internally deposited. External radiation originates from sources external to a particular organism. Weakly penetrating radiations, such as low-energy photons, electrons, and α particles, are of little health concern when originating from external sources but can be of great concern when originating from sources deposited internally. Note that classification as electromagnetic versus particulate, charged versus uncharged, and sparsely versus densely ionizing refers to intrinsic physical properties. However, classification as external versus internal depends only on the happenstance of source location and is not an intrinsic property of radiation.

Another extrinsic classification is that of source or method of production. Here one may separate radiation into three broad categories of extraterrestrial, terrestrial, and human-made. We are already familiar with the first category as cosmic radiation and those radiations arising from cosmic ray interactions. The second category encompasses all radiation arising from the decay of radioisotopes occurring or produced naturally in the environment. The first two categories together constitute natural background radiation. Human-made radiation, which was comparatively rare only 50 years ago, encompasses artificially produced radioisotopes such as those from nuclear weapons testing or reactor wastes, radiation for medical diagnosis and treatment, and a wide variety of radiations used in research and production.

In summary, a short answer to the question posed by the title of this chapter may be attempted in the following manner. Radiation is electromagnetic or particulate energy emitted or produced as the consequence of electron motion, radioactive decay, or atomic and nuclear interactions. Ionizing radiation is that radiation having sufficient energy to produce positive and negative charges directly or indirectly when it interacts with matter. As with many "simple" definitions of complex subjects, this definition contains many terms equally, if not more, complex than the one it purports to define. Like the aroma of a good meal, it conveys a feeling for the subject that should stimulate, rather than satisfy, the appetite.

REFERENCES

1. *Oxford English Dictionary.* London, Oxford University Press, 1961.
2. *Random House Dictionary of the English Language.* New York, Random House, 1973.

2.

Benefits of Radiation

Glenn V. Dalrymple
Max L. Baker and John C. Holder

Radiation-based diagnostic studies involve several types of situations. These situations can be characterized as those in which radiation is absolutely essential, those in which radiation is very useful but perhaps not absolutely necessary, those in which the use of radiation is questionable, and those in which radiation is usually not needed. This chapter presents examples of each of these categories.

RADIATION ABSOLUTELY ESSENTIAL

Serendipity
Serendipity means "the faculty of finding valuable or agreeable things not sought for." As an example, consider the individual for whom a routine x-ray film of the chest is made in the course of employment. On that film he or she is found to have a very small pulmonary nodule that leads to a further work-up, surgery, and the cure of a lung cancer. While this individual certainly received an immeasurable benefit from radiation, the benefit should be considered serendipitous because the x-ray film of the chest was not directed toward finding the lung cancer. The cancer was found "by accident."

Screening Programs
Screening programs represent a step up from blind accident in that large populations of asymptomatic persons are studied with a specific goal in mind. In years past, extensive screening programs were essential for the detection and management of tuberculosis. Currently mammography represents the most popular radiation-based screening program. As discussed in Chapter 12, mammography has great value for diagnosis of occult cancer of the breast.

7

At the same time, mammography is associated with some potential risk. Certainly many lives will be saved if the diagnosis of occult malignancy in the breast can be made and the cancers treated before they become disseminated. On the other hand, there is a small but finite risk of inducing cancer in the normal patient participating in a screening program. As demonstrated in Chapter 12, the benefits outweigh the risks of mammography in many patients, but not in all.

RADIATION NOT ABSOLUTELY NECESSARY

Subdural Hematoma Found by CT Scanning
In unconscious patients with significant subdural hematomas (i.e., intracranial blood between the brain and the skull), the recovery rate exceeds 50 percent if fewer than 6 hours elapse between the time of injury and the time the hematoma is drained. When untreated for a longer period, the recovery rate decreases considerably. The computed tomography (CT) scanner permits the diagnosis of hematoma to be made in a noninvasive manner. If a CT scanner is not available, the diagnosis can still be made by arteriography, wherein a radiopaque contrast medium is injected into an artery and a series of radiographs made. Arteriography, as well as CT scanning, requires radiation. While there is some risk associated with the puncturing of an artery with a needle and the injection of a radiopaque contrast medium, the risk is much less than that associated with leaving the hematoma undrained. Certainly, a blind surgical procedure could be performed when a hematoma is suspected, but the risk of this surgery would be many times greater than that for a diagnostic x-ray procedure. This risk would be particularly troublesome if the presence of a hematoma were only suspected and the clinical indications were not very strong. In the unconscious patient with a subdural hematoma, therefore, radiation may not be absolutely necessary to make the diagnosis, but certainly it is extremely helpful to the patient to have x-ray procedures available.

Unstable Fracture of the Cervical Spine
If the diagnosis of unstable fracture of the cervical spine is not made, the patient is at risk to sever the spinal cord as a result of movement. This would result in either paralysis or death. Consequently, making the diagnosis of an unstable fracture and providing appropriate immobilization are absolutely essential to the patient's well-being. Without the use of radiographs, the diagnosis of such a fracture is extremely difficult to make, and the patient is at risk with regard to the effects of transection of the cord. Radiation therefore provides a definite benefit to the patient.

Ureteral Calculus with an Obstructed Ureter

A patient with this disorder usually experiences severe back pain radiating into the groin. While this clinical picture is frequently characteristic of the disorder, and laboratory signs such as hematuria are usually present, proper management of the patient requires visualization of the stone and determination of the degree of ureteral obstruction, followed by movement of the calculus with time. Left untreated, a totally obstructed ureter may cause destruction of the kidney, and partial obstruction may cause repeated episodes of infection and eventual kidney damage. Without the availability of diagnostic radiologic procedures, the physician would be forced to rely on clinical and laboratory evidence alone, and many unnecessary surgical procedures would be performed. In addition, the likelihood of kidney loss or damage would increase because the clinical signs are not sufficiently reliable to allow the differentiation of patients who need immediate surgery from those who will eventually pass the calculus spontaneously.

Obstructed Cystic Duct on a Nuclear Scan

All physicians are familiar with the patient with acute pain in the right upper quadrant of the abdomen. One of the most important components of the differential diagnosis associated with this clinical presentation is acute cholecystitis secondary to blockage of the cystic duct. This component can be studied very effectively by means of a radioisotope-labeled compound, $^{99m}Tc - N_1\alpha - (p - isopropylacetanilide) - iminodiacetic\ acid$ ($^{99m}Tc - PIPIDA$), which is extracted from the blood by the liver and excreted into the biliary system. Visualization of the gallbladder in this nuclear medicine procedure means that the cystic duct is open, while nonvisualization frequently means that the duct is obstructed by a stone. If an ultrasound examination indicates that the patient has stones in the gallbladder, the combination of clinical signs (obstructed cystic duct and stones in the gallbladder) virtually assures the diagnosis of acute cholecystitis. If the physician were forced to rely on clinical signs alone, surgical delays would occur that would result in gallbladder ruptures. Such ruptures would cause increased mortality and morbidity compared with operation before rupture.

Atherosclerotic Disease of the Coronary Arteries

Coronary artery revascularization procedures are being performed with increasing frequency throughout the world. While there is continued debate about the overall value of this procedure with respect to long-term mortality, many patients state that they experience an improvement in the quality of life after the procedure. Without the identification of the specific diseased arteries by means of coronary arteriography, revascularization procedures would be greatly hampered and perhaps could not be performed at all.

Other Examples

A large number of other beneficial uses of radiation could be discussed. Among these uses are demonstration of pneumothorax in patients with respiratory distress syndrome, diagnosis of a ruptured aorta in a motorcycle accident victim, detection of a ruptured esophagus (Boerhaave's syndrome), demonstration of occult radial head fractures after injury to the elbow, identification of a perforated viscus, and so on. In all these instances, x-ray procedures are not absolutely critical to the diagnosis since, sooner or later, the disorder will become clinically apparent. Without diagnostic radiologic studies, however, the patient would probably be dead or severely maimed before an adequate diagnosis of the condition could be made.

RADIATION QUESTIONABLE

Diagnosis of Acute Appendicitis

The clinical presentation of acute appendicitis is generally sufficient for a diagnosis to be made without the use of radiographs. Occasionally, however, a barium enema can be very helpful by demonstrating the filling or nonfilling of the appendix, with the latter condition associated with appendicitis.

Repeated Upper GI Series in a Patient with Known Peptic Ulcer

Once the diagnosis of peptic ulcer is made, particularly in a patient who has had symptoms for a number of years, repeated upper gastrointestinal (GI) series are usually of limited value. If upper GI bleeding develops, endoscopy (gastroscopy) may provide more benefit than repeated barium studies.

Repeated X-Ray Studies of an Uncomplicated Healing Fracture

Experienced orthopedic surgeons who feel comfortable with the immediate postreduction and casting status of a patient do not require a large number of x-ray examinations to follow the course of healing of an uncomplicated fracture. Relatively frequent filming is helpful only in such instances as a fracture that has been a compound break or in which there is a suggestion of nonunion.

RADIATION USUALLY NOT NEEDED

Most Psychiatric Illnesses

Relatively few psychiatric illnesses have a radiologic manifestation. Predictably, then, patients admitted to hospitals with psychiatric disorders have relatively few radiographs made. As one exception, the demonstration of normal pressure hydrocephalus by CT scanning may be beneficial. For this disorder the triad of dementia, incontinence, and ataxia may be treated by ventricular shunting. Earlier, radionuclide cisternograms were used to demonstrate the presence of this condition. More recently, CT scanning has replaced the cisternogram. On occasion, the patient who actually has hyperthyroidism is mistakenly thought to have a psychiatric disorder. Appropriate laboratory diagnostic studies, including radioiodine uptake (a radiation application), will identify the presence of hyper-thyroidism.

Most Ophthalmologic Conditions

The patient with a nontraumatic ophthalmologic disorder generally does not require radiation-based diagnostic studies. CT scanning can be helpful in localizing metallic foreign bodies in the eye and in identifying tumors and other destructive processes involving the eye and orbital contents. In general, however, radiation is not used extensively in the management of ophthalmologic conditions.

Most Dermatologic Disorders

Most conditions of the skin do not require the use of radiation for purposes of diagnosis. However, radiation is occasionally helpful in patients having a dermatologic manifestation of a systemic disorder. For example, psoriasis may be associated with extensive arthritis, particularly of the hands, in addition to skin lesions.

CONCLUSION

Selected clinical examples have been represented in which radiation is of great benefit, of limited benefit, or essentially of no benefit to the patient. When psychiatric, ophthalmologic, and dermatologic disorders are excluded, most disease states have some form of presentation in radiation-based diagnostic examinations. As the patient and physician become better informed of the benefits and risks of these studies, they will be better directed to solving a diagnostic problem while reducing the radiation burden to the patient.

3.

Overview of the Hazards of Low-Level Exposure to Radiation

E. Russell Ritenour

The harmful effects of high levels of radiation are well known from studies of such groups as the atom bomb survivors, radium dial painters, and pioneer radiologists who used (by today's standards) primitive equipment and were unaware of the hazards of radiation. Most people are familiar with the term "radiation sickness." This is a short-term, or immediate, health effect technically known as the acute radiation syndrome (ARS). One symptom of ARS is the nausea and vomiting that occur shortly after a whole-body dose of a few hundred rem delivered over a very short period of time. It may be followed within a few weeks by diarrhea, emaciation, loss of hair, fever, sore throat, subcutaneous bleeding, and bleeding from body orifices. Approximately half of those receiving a dose of 500 rem will die within about 30 days. Below 1,000-rem doses, deaths that occur will be attributable to failure of the hematopoietic system. Infection and bleeding will be the direct cause of death within 1 month. For doses between 1,000 and 10,000 rem, the gastrointestinal (GI) system will be severely affected, causing death within days resulting from ulceration and bleeding in the GI tract. Doses above 10,000 rem will immediately affect cells of the nervous system, bringing death within hours. Amounts of radiation sufficient to cause such immediate and devastating health effects might be encountered from nuclear weapons exposure or severe industrial accidents. We may think of these cases as analogous to overdoses of some strong chemical agent.

In this chapter we are concerned with low-level radiation, doses of ionizing radiation that are ten to thousands of times smaller than those required to contract ARS. Low-level radiation may be defined as an absorbed dose of 10 rem or less delivered over a short period of time. A larger dose delivered over a long period of time, for instance, 50 rem in 10 years, may also be considered low level. The definition is purposely loose so as to cover a wide variety of sources of radiation exposure, such as natural background (100 mrem/year), occupational exposures ($<$ 5 rem/year), and medical applications, such as diagnostic radiography ($<$ 1 rem). Low-level radiation exposure does not produce ARS.

The health effects that may be of concern in regard to low-level radiation are its long-term sequelae. Studies of survivors of high-level radiation exposure (both human and laboratory animals) have indicated that there are three health effects that should be examined at low levels of exposure: induction of cancer, birth abnormalities (from irradiation in utero), and genetic effects. No other long-term effects of low-level exposure have been conclusively demonstrated in animals or humans.

INDUCTION OF CANCER

It is known that large amounts of radiation will significantly increase the incidence of cancer in a population. At low doses of radiation, however, it is difficult to detect radiation-induced cancer because (1) the number of radiation-induced cases is small and (2) cancer from natural causes is so prevalent a disease. It is estimated that the natural incidence of fatal cancer for the U.S. population is 16%.[1] The incidence of nonfatal cancer is also about 16%, so that the likelihood is about 1:3 that a person will experience cancer, either fatal or nonfatal in his or her lifetime. Radiation produces no unique types of cancer but will, when given in large quantities, yield an increase over the natural incidence of many types of cancer. How then can we discover the contribution that small amounts of radiation make to the risk that a person will contract fatal cancer? One way is to study populations that have received large amounts of radiation, such as the 100,000 or so survivors of the atomic bomb blasts in Hiroshima and Nagasaki. This group was exposed to doses of hundreds of rem. Those who survived ARS were then susceptible to the long-term effects of radiation. In a population of this size we can estimate the number of fatal cancers that would have occurred had there been no radiation exposure. We can then study the number of fatal cancers that actually occurred and determine the difference. Among the atom bomb survivors it has been estimated that there have been approximately 200 excess cancer deaths to date.[2] While the tremendous social, psychological, and environmental upheaval suffered by this group may have played some role in this increase in fatal cancer, it is reasonable to attribute most of it to the radiation exposure.

At this point we may ask the question: Would a population that has been exposed to half as much radiation as the atom bomb survivors have half as many excess cancers? How about a population that has received 1/100 as much radiation? As the radiation dose becomes smaller, the number of excess

fatal cancers also becomes smaller, until it is difficult to see any difference between an irradiated and a control population. At low-dose levels, studies of
actual populations become inconclusive. Experiments can be done with large
populations of animals, which have much shorter life-spans than humans and
therefore yield better statistical results, but one must then make assumptions
as to the relevance of animal studies to human populations. One way to approach the problem is to use reliable data to determine a dose–effect relationship for humans at high doses and then to extrapolate the effect to low doses.
This procedure is illustrated by curves a–c in Figure 1. The shape of the curve
in the high-dose region of the graph is well known from studies of the atom
bomb survivors. But in the low-dose region of the graph, the shape of the
curve must be inferred from less conclusive human studies or from animal experiments. On the basis of such evidence, most scientists would consider curve
c to represent an extreme overestimate of the effects of small amounts of
radiation. There is considerable evidence to support curve b as the correct

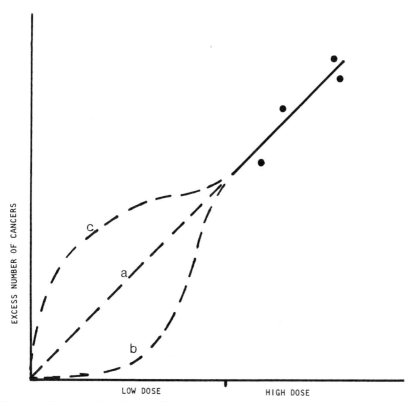

Figure 1. Extrapolation of dose-effect data.

representation.[3] Since there is some uncertainty, most scientists accept curve a, known as the linear model, as an upper limit of the actual dose-effect relationship. It is therefore a conservative estimate, or overestimate, of the actual risk. According to the linear model, if the dose is decreased to half, the effect (i.e., number of fatal cancers) will be decreased by half. We will assume that the linear model is correct for the purposes of this discussion.

On the basis of the linear model, it has been calculated that in a population of one million receiving a dose of 1 rem delivered in a short period of time, 100–200 excess cancer deaths will occur over the lifetimes within the population[1]. This result should be compared with the 160,000 cancer deaths that will occur in the population in the absence of this "extra" radiation. To extrapolate further, natural background radiation, about 0.1 rem/year, could be said to cause 1–2 percent of the 160,000 fatal cancers that occur "naturally." We can attempt to determine, or at least to verify, this number experimentally. Background radiation levels vary in different parts of the world. Studies have been done to compare cancer incidence in areas in which background radiation is low to the incidence in regions of high background. These studies have been done in the United States, China, Brazil, and India. In all cases, the results have been inconclusive[4-8]; that is, even though some regions of the United States and other countries have significantly more background radiation than do other regions (dose rates in parts of India approach 1.3 rem/year), there is no detectable increase in the incidence of cancer. So there is an apparent discrepancy between theoretical predictions and experimental results. One theory that might explain this discrepancy is that natural background is not as hazardous to humankind as one might expect, possibly because humankind has evolved for millenia in the presence of this small amount of radiation. Therefore, life on this planet is biologically compatible with amounts of radiation that are not much greater than a few tenths of rem[3]. Perhaps a more plausible explanation is that other factors influence cancer incidence more than does background radiation. In any case, the linear model appears, on the basis of these studies, to overestimate the risk.

Studies have also been done of populations exposed to low levels of radiation beyond background as a result of occupational exposure, medical procedures, and exposure to atomic weapons fallout.[1,2,9] A small number of scientists believe that these studies demonstrate a significant increase in cancer incidence over that of populations not exposed to these "extra" sources of radiation and that this increase is even greater than the linear model predicts. The report released in 1980 of the committee of the National Academy of Sciences charged with the study of low-level radiation effects states the following[1]:

> None of these studies was considered by the Committee to constitute reliable evidence at present for use in risk estimation for various reasons, in-

cluding inadequate sample size in some instances, inadequate statistical analysis, and unconfirmed results.

BIRTH ABNORMALITIES

The embryo is known to be affected by high-level radiation. There are two main reasons for this effect. First, it has been known for many years that rapidly dividing cells are especially radiosensitive.[10] The embryonic cells fit this description during the early stages of development. Second, since the embryo is composed of a small number of cells during the very early stages of life, each cell is vital to the development of the fetus.

The effects of high-level radiation on the embryo are embryonic, fetal or neonatal death, intrauterine growth retardation (IUGR), and congenital malformation.[11] The effects of low-level radiation on the embryo are not as well documented. One reason for this lack of documentation is that in 4-6 percent of all live births in the United States, some type of abnormality is present. The abnormalities known to be produced by high levels of radiation are no different in kind from those that occur spontaneously. Another difficulty is the natural genetic and environmental variability of human populations. Because of these difficulties, the influence of low-level radiation on birth abnormalities is estimated, as is cancer induction, from animal experiments and by extrapolation from studies of populations exposed to high levels of radiation. If the irradiation occurs over a short period of time, it is speculated that the effects on the embryo are dependent on the stage of development at which the irradiation occurs.[9] Effects such as malformation appear to be more pronounced when exposure occurs during the period of formation of major organ systems (second through ninth week in the human). In any case, the risk of harm caused by low-level radiation is small. A recent review of the literature on this subject[12] indicates that 1 rem delivered to the embryo before the ninth week would not increase the chance of gross congenital malformations, IUGR, or death. Some researchers believe that the embryo is more susceptible to radiation-induced leukemia than is the adult. Estimates of the risk of leukemia resulting from a 1-rem dose to the embryo range from 1: 1,000[13] to 1: 10 million.[12] Background radiation of about 60 mrem or 0.2 mrem/day is therefore an insignificant health hazard with respect to the embryo. This finding has been demonstrated in epidemiologic studies.[14]

Fetal irradiation can occur during medical procedures. Unfortunately, most women are not aware that they are pregnant during the very early period of pregnancy when the fetus is most sensitive to radiation. For this reason, care is taken during medical procedures involving ionizing radiation to minimize the chance that pregnant women might receive appreciable amounts of radiation to the fetal area. Data from the atom bomb survivors suggest that measurable damage such as microcephaly or small head size does not occur at doses of < 50 rem.[15] Even though diagnostic procedures rarely result in absorbed doses to the fetal area of more than a fraction of 1 rem, caution is observed. For these reasons, diagnostic radiologic procedures do not normally constitute a health hazard to the embryo.

GENETIC EFFECTS

Serious genetic disorders are common, since they occur in more than 10 percent of all live births in the United States.[1] Animal experiments show that radiation has a limited effect on genetic disorders. But at this time it is difficult to determine the impact of infrequent mutations on generations far into the future.[15] The problem has received considerable attention, however, and it is safe to say that the mutational effects of radiation are at least as well understood as those of any chemical mutagen in the environment.

To understand the effect of radiation on the incidence of genetic disorders it is important to first understand the magnitude of the problem in the absence of radiation. Although a comprehensive list of human genetic disorders is yet to be completed, some of the best data to date have been compiled by the Committee on the Biological Effects of Ionizing Radiation (BEIR), a committee of the National Academy of Sciences.[1] Incidence figures given below are from this source.

Genetic disorders can be classified according to their mode of inheritance. Disorders involving individual genes might be dominant or recessive. If dominant, the first generation of offspring will probably be affected after mutation occurs in a parent. Various bone disorders and certain types of muscular dystrophy exhibit dominant patterns of inheritance. One percent of the population suffers from a severe dominant disorder. In recessive mutations, many generations may pass before offspring exhibit symptoms of a disorder. Two persons having the recessive genetic trait would have to mate before that trait would have even a small chance of being expressed in the offspring. It is also possible that a mutant recessive gene will be lost from the population before it ever encounters another like itself. Recessive gene traits are responsible for more than 600 diseases.[16] A few, such as sickle cell anemia and cystic fibrosis, are common but most are quite rare.

Many genetic disorders, such as cleft palate, follow neither dominant nor recessive inheritance patterns. These mutations exhibit "irregular" inheritance patterns and make up the bulk (90 percent) of the genetic burden of human populations.

Some types of genetic disorders are caused by the breaking and rearrangement of chromosomes. These types of aberrations often result in early embryonic death and are therefore not often passed on to succeeding generations. These disorders affect fewer than 0.1 percent of the population, result-ing in problems such as Down's syndrome. Other more subtle genetic effects have been found in experiments with the fruit fly, *Drosophila melangaster*, to be among the most frequent types of genetic abnormalities.[1] These types of disorders result in very mild (nearly undetectable) effects, such as a 1 percent reduction in the probability of survival from egg to adult stage.

In experimental animals, radiation has been associated with dominant, recessive, and irregular types of genetic mutations. The amount of chromo-somal aberration has been shown to be small[17] compared with the other types. Unfortunately, it is difficult to demonstrate the more subtle types of viability disorders in species other than the very short-lived fruit fly. The population size and time required to demonstrate a trait that can only be uncovered sta-tistically over many generations are prohibitively large for mammalian studies.

To date no conclusive data exist to demonstrate genetic damage in humans caused by low-level radiation. Studies of A-bomb survivors have shown no relationship between radiation exposure and harmful genetic ef-fects such as birth defects or increased infant mortality in successive genera-tions. This finding suggests that there is no great effect, at least on the first and possibly the second generation. Therefore, dominant-type disorders do not appear to be readily produced by radiation. The risk of genetic effects of low-level ionizing radiation has been calculated by the BEIR committee on the basis of animal data, such as the incidence of radiation-induced skeletal mutations in mice. According to this source, if each generation receives one additional rem of radiation to the gonads, 0.006-0.110 percent of the popula-tion will incur radiation-induced genetic malformations after many genera-tions have passed. This range represents the total impact of the different types of genetic disorders discussed in this section and should be compared with the current "natural" incidence of more than 10 percent.

COMPARATIVE RISKS

Most of the preceding discussions have involved calculations of the risk of low-level radiation based on extrapolation from high levels. Many studies of actual populations, such as the studies of high and low natural background regions mentioned previously, do not find the magnitude of health effects called for by the linear dose–effect hypothesis. One recent study suggests that environmental chemicals, especially sulfur and nitrogen dioxide and par-ticulate sulfate, have more adverse effects on health than does background radiation.[18] In any case, there is not yet significant experimental evidence that the linear hypothesis extends to low levels. In all likelihood, therefore, the linear hypothesis represents an over-estimate of risk which, for the pur-

TABLE 1. LOSS OF LIFE EXPECTANCY ATTRIBUTABLE
TO VARIOUS CAUSES

Cause	Days
Cigarette smoking, male	2,250
Heart disease	2,100
Being a coal miner	1,100
Cancer	980
Cigarette smoking, female	800
Stroke	520
Army in Vietnam	400
Motor vehicle accidents	207
Accidents in home	95
Diabetes	95
Drowning	41
Falls	39
Accidents to pedestrians	37
Natural background radiation	8
Medical x-rays	6
Coffee	6
Diet drinks	2

*Adapted from Cohen BL and Lee I-sing: A catalog of risks
Health Phys 1979; 36:720.*

pose of standards-setting in the interest of public health, can be viewed as conservative.

To gain a balanced perspective of the risks associated with low level radiation exposure, it it instructive to consider the risks associated with more familiar occurrences. Perhaps one of the easiest ways to compare these risks is to look at the effect of each on life expectancy.

Because of the incidence of heart disease in the United States, the life expectancy of an average citizen is shortened by 2,100 days, or a little less than 6 years. According to the National Safety Council, about 800,000 deaths per year are currently attributable to heart disease. Motor vehicle accidents shorten life expectancy by 207 days, or 7 months, because of the average age of the 50,000 persons who have vehicle fatalities each year. In Table 1 the loss of life expectancy is attributable to various causes as determined by data obtained from sources such as the U.S. Bureau of Census. As expected, heart disease, cancer, and stroke significantly shorten the life-span of the average American. According to Table 1, a nationwide average exposure of medical x-rays could be expected, according to a widely used National Academy of Sciences dose–effect hypothesis, to shorten the life of an average citizen by no more than 6 days. No statistics support a figure of this size; rather, it represents a "worst-case" estimate.

This conclusion does not take into account any of the benefits of medical x-rays, such as increased life expectancy resulting from early diagnosis of disease. For example, it has been estimated that an x-ray film of the chest saves 5 working days on average.[19] One should also take into account a non-quantifiable result of many medical x-rays, namely the alleviation of pain and suffering. Finally, Table 1 demonstrates that the science of risk analysis has reached the stage at which extremely small hazards can be estimated and, furthermore, that low-level radiation is among the least of the many hazards encountered by modern man.

REFERENCES

1. Committee on the Biological Effects of Ionizing Radiations of the National Academy of Sciences: The Effects on Populations of Exposure to Low Levels of Ionizing Radiation. Washington DC, National Academy Press, 1980, pp 118-181.
2. Problems in Assessing the Cancer Risks of Low-Level Ionizing Radiation Exposure. Report to the Congress of the United States, V1 11. Washington DC, United States General Accounting Office, January 1981, Appendix II.
3. Adler HI: An approach to setting radiation standards. *Health Phys* 1978; 34: 719-720.
4. Friere-Maia A, Friere-Maia DV: Mortality Rates in a Brazilian Area of High Background Radiation. Preliminary analysis based on official records. *Nucl Sci Abst* 22, 38453, 1968.
5. Penna Franca E, et al: Status of investigations in the Brazilian areas of high natural radioactivity. *Health Phys* 1965; 11:699.
6. Mills WA, Youmans HD: Population exposures from natural background radiation in Kerala, India. *Health Phys* 1968; 15:188, abst.
7. Rao KR: Report on Kerala (India), A region with high background radiation. *Nucl Sci* Abst 21, 34672, 1967.
8. High Background Radiation Research Group: China. Health survey in high background radiation areas in China. *Science* 1980; 290:877-880.
9. Miller RW, Mulvihill JJ: Small head size after atomic irradiation. *Teratology* 1976; 14:355-357.
10. Bergonie JA, Tribondeau L: Interpretation of some results of radiotherapy and an attempt at determining a logical technique of treatment. *Radiat Res* 1959; 11:587.
11. Blot WJ, Miller RW: Mental retardation following *in utero* exposure to the atomic bombs of Hiroshima and Nagasaki. *Radiology* 1973; 106:617-619.
12. Brent RL: Radiation teratogenesis, teratogen update. *Teratology* 1980; 21:281-298.
13. Stewart A: The carcinogenic effects of low level radiation. A re-appraisal of epidemiologists methods and observations. *Health Phys* 1973; 24:223-240.
14. Grahm D, Kratchman J: Variation in neonatal death rate and birth weight in the United States and possible relations to environmental radiation, geology and altitude. *Am J Hum Genet* 1963; 15:329-352.
15. Crow JF: How Well Can We Assess Genetic Risk: Not Very. The Lauriston S.

Taylor Lecture Series in Radiation Protection and Measurements, Lecture No 5. Washington DC, National Council on Radiation Protection and Measurements, 1981.

16. McKusick VA: *Mendalian Inheritance in Man: Catalogs of Autosomal Dominant, Autosomal Recessive and X-linked Phenotypes.* ed 5. Baltimore, Johns Hopkins University Press, 1978.

17. Selby PB: Genetic effects of low-level irradiation, in Fullerton GD, et al (eds) *Biological Risks of Medical Irradiations.* Medical Physics Monograph No 5. American Association of Physicists in Medicine, 1980, pp 1–20.

18. Hickey RL, et al: Low level ionizing radiation and human mortality: Multi-regional epidemiological studies. A preliminary report. *Health Phys* 1981; 40:625.

19. Gregg EC: Risk/benefit considerations in radiology, in Fullerton GD, et al (eds) Biological Risks of Medical Irradiations. Medical Physics Monograph No 5. American Association of Physicists in Medicine, 1980, pp 160–176.

4.

Truths and Fallacies Concerning Radiation and Its Effects

Steven R. Wilkins

In childhood we learned many myths about radiation. For example, we were told that people exposed to x-rays would glow in the dark, become radioactive, or, under the proper circumstances, turn into superhumans such as the "Hulk" or "Spiderman." Although these and other childhood myths are not taken seriously, many misconceptions still exist about the effects of ionizing radiation. Does exposure to radiation necessarily imply an ill fate? It is the intent of this chapter to highlight a few of the truths and fallacies concerning radiation and its effects.

One common misconception is that ionizing radiation is capable of creating unique diseases. Artificial or natural sources of radiation do not cause unique diseases or abnormalities. The same kind of genetic mutations produced by radiation can be caused by other mutagenic agents, such as certain drugs, chemicals, or viral infections. Cells of cancers induced by radiation are indistinguishable from cells of cancers induced by other substances or activities in our environment. If an expectant mother receives an abdominal x-ray examination and the child is born with some type of abnormality, it would be impossible to trace it definitely to the x-ray exposure. This lack of identification between cause and effect on an individual basis is one reason that it is extremely difficult for scientists to measure the biological effects of ionizing radiation precisely, particularly for low levels of radiation exposure. What is possible is to estimate roughly the number of additional harmful effects attributable to radiation exposure that might occur over and above the naturally occurring incidences in a given population.

A second misconception is that ionizing radiation from a medical procedure is more hazardous than the disease to be detected or eradicated. The risk of not having an examination is generally much greater than that of the procedure. Few people would dispute that, since its discovery in the late

1890s, the medical use of ionizing radiation has saved millions of lives. Diagnostic x-ray examinations and nuclear medicine procedures help physicians diagnose a large number of illnesses and internal conditions, including heart disease, infections, ulcers, tumors, cysts, arthritis, blood clots, and lacerations, that might otherwise remain hidden or obscure. Diagnosis of a disease enables the physician to apply the proper course of treatment quickly. If detected, a disease such as cancer can be treated before further damage occurs. The risks from exposure are offset by the tangible benefit a cancer patient may receive from treatment. If the examination detects no abnormalities, however, the benefit is less readily seen, since any patient undergoing a radiologic procedure may incur some risk of long-term radiation effects. Even a negative finding has merit in that it allows the physician to look for other suspected causes. Conversely, without a radiologic examination there is an increased probability of missing information that would cause the physician to alter the patient's course of treatment.

Induction of cancer and genetic damage are of principal concern to populations exposed to low levels of ionizing radiation. The best educated estimate for the lifetime risk of cancer mortality induced by radiation is approximately 77-226 excess cancer deaths per million persons per rad.[1] Although doses may vary considerably, none of the more comprehensive types of diagnostic radiologic procedures involves doses of more than a few rads.[2] If we assume an effective dose of 1 rad and the average of the risk estimates, the lifetime risk estimate translates into approximately 151 cancer deaths per one million persons (a risk of about 1:6,600). Also, exposure of the reproductive organs (gonads) is thought to increase the chance, although only very slightly, of passing on defective genes to future generations. In the first generation, it is estimated that 1 rad of parental exposure will result in an increase of 5-75 additional serious genetic disorders per million liveborn offsprings.[1] The possible genetic risk should be included with the cancer risk in assessing the total radiation impact.

In the treatment of diseases with ionizing radiation, the doses can be many hundreds of rads where destruction of the cancer cells is desired; irradiation of some normal healthy tissue is unavoidable. The risks associated with therapeutic doses of radiation, which might become manifest several years later, are correspondingly higher than risks associated with diagnostic procedures. During the mid-1930s to the mid-1950s many patients were treated with large exposures of x-rays (approximately 250-2,500 roentgens) to the spinal marrow for a progressively disabling arthritic disease of the spine. Of the approximately 14,000 patients treated, about 60 developed leukemia some years later, as opposed to perhaps seven cases that would have been expected in the same number of people not irradiated.[3] This is not a particularly large risk when weighed against the chronic pain of a disabled patient.

There are some situations in which the benefit derived from a procedure is questionable. These may include x-ray films required for employment for legal protection of employers and x-ray films ordered because of the physician's concern for potential malpractice suits. In both cases, the likelihood of a medical gain to the patient appears doubtful. Unnecessary procedures providing little or no benefit to the patient should be avoided. By no means should a patient avoid x-ray films if any significant medical benefit can be gained, however.

Another misconception is that exposure arising from diagnostic procedures during pregnancy is likely to lead to a deformed child. According to the best available knowledge, malformations are unlikely to occur in the unborn children whose mothers undergo radiologic examinations. Evidence indicates that the most sensitive stage for the production of malformations is between the second and tenth weeks of pregnancy (first trimester). For any individual case, the increased risk of an abnormality from doses below 10 rads received at any stage of pregnancy is thought to be very small when compared with the naturally occurring incidence of congenital defects (4-6 percent). Only for doses above 15 rad is the risk of malformations considered significantly increased above control levels.[4] An extraordinary number of x-ray procedures would have to occur for such large fetal doses to accumulate. Therefore, the exposure of the fetus to ionizing radiation from diagnostic procedures would very rarely be cause, in itself, for terminating a pregnancy.[4]

It is very unlikely that exposure to medical procedures using ionizing radiation will lead to an ill fate. According to most radiation experts, the total health hazard that may exist for populations receiving occupational or medical exposures to ionizing radiation is slight at most and compares favorably with other potential hazards to which people are regularly exposed, including motor vehicles, electric power, and swimming.

REFERENCES

1. National Research Council, Advisory Committee on the Biological Effects of Ionizing Radiation: The Effects on Populations of Exposure to Low Levels of Ionizing Radiations. Washington DC, National Academy of Sciences, 1980.

2. National Council on Radiation Protection and Measurements: Basic Radiation Protection Criteria. Report No 39. Washington DC, National Council on Radiation Protection and Measurements, 1971.

3. Court-Brown WR, Doll R: Mortality from cancer and other causes after radiotherapy for ankylosing spondylitis. Br Med J 1965; 2:1327-1332.

4. National Council on Radiation Protection and Measurements. Medical radiation exposure of pregnant and potentially pregnant women. Report No. 54. Washington, DC, National Council of Radiation Protection and Measurement, 1977.

5.

Sources of Low-Level Radiation Effects Data

Steven R. Wilkins

There is an extensive body of knowledge and experience on the biologic effects of ionizing radiation. In fact, there is probably more scientific evidence on the health risks of radiation than on any other potentially hazardous agent. Despite this abundance of data, considerable controversy among radiation experts still exists, contributing to public confusion and fear concerning the health hazards that might exist for populations receiving low doses of radiation, such as those received in diagnostic radiologic procedures and occupational exposures.

To understand the controversy and avoid gross misconceptions of radiation risks, as occurred during the Three Mile Island incident, for example, it is helpful to review the sources of radiation effects data. This chapter gives major emphasis to the human evidence on the carcinogenic effects of ionizing radiation; evidence on other somatic effects and genetic effects is discussed in other presentations in this volume. It is the intent of this chapter to help provide a foundation upon which a reasonable understanding of radiation risks can be developed.

It is known that radiation in large amounts does cause an increase in cancer in humans. The chief sources of human data providing this evidence are epidemiologic studies involving populations exposed to relatively high levels of radiation either medically, occupationally, or from atomic bombs. The largest of the study populations are the survivors of the 1945 atomic bomb explosions at Hiroshima and Nagasaki. Studies of the mortality of A-bomb survivors exposed at all dose levels have confirmed the carcinogenic effect of ionizing radiation with respect to leukemia, breast cancer, and lung cancer, and more recently to cancer of the esophagus, stomach, and urinary organs, as well as the lymphomas.[1] A study has also confirmed that the carcinogenic effect, measured in terms of relative risk, is highest among those under age 10 at the time of the bomb explosion.[2] The minimal latent period for most of the carcinogenic effects was under 15 years. Absolute risk estimates of mortality from all causes of deaths for both cities averaged 3.89 excess deaths per million persons/year/rad for the period 1950-1974.

Early human evidence of occupationally related carcinogenic effects of radiation has been based primarily on the experience of pioneering scientists, radiologists, x-ray technicians, dentists, miners, and radium dial painters. Largely unaware of the hazards of radiation, and hence taking few precautions, many of these early practitioners and workers died from leukemia and cancer of the skin, bone, and lung. Dentists, for example, often developed skin lesions on their fingers from repeatedly holding dental films in their patients' mouths, and miners often developed lung cancer from inhaling air-borne radioactivity underground. These early occupational exposures are of interest, since they have shown increased mortality rates over that of the general population or their counterparts.[3-5] Generally they have not, however, yielded reliable quantitative data.

The third major source of human evidence arises from studies involving patients exposed to radiation for medical purposes. Increased incidence of thyroid cancer, for example, has been demonstrated in infants with respiratory distress who were diagnosed as having enlarged thymus glands and who were subsequently treated with therapeutic doses (200-600 rad) of x-rays to that area.[6] The linear risk estimate is 2.5 excess thyroid cancer cases per million persons/year/rad.

Increased incidence of breast cancer has been demonstrated in women receiving high doses of radiation to the chest. One survey involved women treated for tuberculosis by artificial pneumothorax, a procedure consisting of collapsing and later reinflating the affected lung with the assistance of fluoroscopy.[7] The women in this study, living 10 years or more following the first fluoroscopic exposure, were estimated to have a breast cancer risk of 6.2 radiation-induced breast cancer cases per million women/year/rad. On average, each woman received a cumulative breast dose of approximately 150 rad. Another study showing a somewhat similar increase in breast cancer incidence (8-10 excess breast cancer cases per million women/year/rad) involved a group of women treated for postpartum mastitis, inflammation of the breast, after childbirth.[8]

Perhaps the single greatest source of data related to the health effects of exposure to medical radiation is the long-term epidemiologic study of patients exposed to therapeutic radiation for treatment of ankylosing spondylitis, a progressively disabling arthritic disease of the spine. During the mid-1930s to the mid 1950s in Great Britain and Northern Ireland, these patients were treated with large exposures of x-rays (approximately 250-2,500 roentgens to the spinal marrow). It was not until the late 1950s, however, that an unusually high rate of leukemia became apparent among these people. Of the approximately 14,000 patients treated, leukemia developed in about 60, whereas perhaps seven cases would have been expected in the same number of people not irradiated.[9]

Data from the above studies and others, which generally involved doses of $\geq$ 50 rad, contribute to an impressive accumulation of evidence demonstrating the carcinogenic effects of ionizing radiation. As an alternative to using high-dose data and mathematical models to predict excess cancers that may be induced by low doses of radiation, some scientists have attempted to study directly populations that have received low exposures to radiation. It certainly would be preferred to assess any hazard involved with radiation on the basis of realistic human data acquired at the actual dose levels of concern. Several recent controversial studies of populations exposed to low levels of ionizing radiation that indicate increased cancer incidence over the expected natural incidence include (1) the Oxford survey, which found an increased risk of leukemia and other cancers among children who had been irradiated in utero as a result of pelvic x-ray examination of the mother[10,11]; (2) a study on employees at the Hanford Nuclear Facility, who received occupational exposures during the period 1944–1972[12,13]; (3) a claim concerning increased infant mortality from 1976 Chinese atomic bomb fallout[14]; (4) 1977 and 1979 reports claiming supersensitivity of certain types of subjects to diagnostic x-rays[15,16]; and (5) a 1979 report on Utah children who may have been exposed to fallout from atmospheric nuclear weapon tests in Nevada between 1951 and 1958.[17]

Allegations of these studies and others, which have attempted to demonstrate deleterious effects in humans in the low-dose range, have been subject to serious criticism or offset by other studies with negative results and, therefore, remain unproved.[18-25] In the study of Court-Brown et al,[18] for example, follow-up of 39,166 liveborn children whose mothers were known to have had abdominal or pelvic irradiation during their pregnancy showed no excess of leukemia. Similarly, in another study, no significant excess of mortality from leukemia or other cancers was found of 1,292 children exposed prenatally in 1945 to the atomic bombs in Hiroshima and Nagasaki.[19] The results of both studies are in disagreement with the findings of Stewart and her colleagues at Oxford.

A number of recent papers have attempted to compare cancer rates among populations exposed to various background radiation levels, that is, very low dose levels. The results of a study by Archer[26] published in 1978, indicate a link between increased cosmic radiation levels and increased cancer deaths. Archer believes that as much as approximately 40–50 percent of all cancer is a result of exposure to background radiation. In contrast, Frigerio and Stowe[27] found an inverse relationship between background radiation levels and cancer death rates in the United States. It seems likely that effects of differences in background radiation on cancer induction are so small that other factors related to cancer might be dominating.[22]

In addition to carcinogenic risks, genetic risks are of principal concern to populations exposed to ionizing radiation at low doses. No genetic effects of ionizing radiation (i.e., effects transmitted to descendants) have been clearly demonstrated in human populations.[22] Even among the offspring of the Japanese atomic bomb survivors, for example, no significant effect of parental exposure on child survival has appeared.[28] Animal experimentation, with the most relevant genetic data coming from experiments involving mice, remains the primary source of data for estimation of possible genetic risks to humans.

Estimates of the genetic effects of radiation are based largely on data collected in mice using either the specific-locus method or the approach of looking for genetic damage to the skeleton. Studies on mouse populations using the specific-locus method have provided a considerable pool of information concerning the factors affecting the frequency of mutations, such as dose rate, fractionation, sex, and cell stage.[22] In mouse spermatogonia, for example, there is evidence that the frequency of mutations drops as the exposure rate is lowered from 90 R/min to 0.8 R/min; below that level to even 0.0007 R/min, there is no further reduction in genetic effect.[29] This observation is the basis for the belief that there is no threshold exposure rate in the male and that the frequency of mutation at low exposures is linear. The second method is based on work that has shown that high-dose irradiation (gamma radiation of 100 R − 500 R, delivered at 60 R/min with a 24-hour interval between fractions) induces a fairly high frequency of dominant mutations that causes skeletal abnormalities.[30] The estimates arrived at by the two methods are in good agreement. In the first generation, the genetic risk estimate to humans for 1 rem of parental exposure is 5-75 additional serious genetic disorders per million liveborn offspring.[22]

To date, it is not possible to predict a precise number of cancers or genetic disorders that may be caused by low doses of radiation such as those received in diagnostic radiologic procedures and in occupational exposures. Exact risk estimates are probably not achievable until basic mechanisms by which ionizing radiation caused cancers are better understood. So far, evidence indicates that carcinogenic and genetic risks are small compared with the naturally occurring incidence of cancers and serious genetic defects.

REFERENCES

1. Beebe GW, Kato H, Land CE: Studies of the mortality of A-bomb survivors. 6. Mortality and radiation dose, 1950-1974. *Radiat Res* 1978;75: 138-201.
2. Jablon S, Kato H: Studies of the mortality of A-bomb survivors. 5. Radiation dose and mortality, 1950-1970. *Radiat Res* 1972;50: 649-698.
3. Polednak AP, Stehney AF, Rowland RE: Mortality among women first em-

ployed before 1930 in the U.S. radium dial-painting industry. *Am J Epidemiol* 1978; 107: 179-195.

4. Matanoski GM, Seltzer R. Sartwell PE, et al: The current mortality rates of radiologists and other physician specialists: deaths from all causes and from cancer. *Am J Epidemiol*, 1975;101: 188-193.

5. Archer VE, Gillam JD. Wagoner JK: Respiratory disease mortality among uranium miners. *Ann NY Acad Sci* 1972;271: 280-293.

6. Hempelmann LH, Hall WJ, Phillips M, et al: Neoplasms in persons treated with x-rays in infancy: Fourth survey in 20 years. *J Natl Cancer Inst* 1975;55: 519-530.

7. Boice JD Jr, Rosenstein M, Trout ED: Estimation of breast doses and breast cancer risk associated with repeated fluoroscopic chest examinations of women with tuberculosis. *Pediat Res* 1978;73: 373-390.

8. Store RE, Hempelmann LH, Kowaluk E, et al: Breast neoplasms in women treated with x-rays for acute postpartum mastitis. *J Natl Cancer Inst* 1977;59: 813-822.

9. Court-Brown WR, Doll R: Mortality from cancer and other causes after radiotherapy for ankylosing spondylitis. *Br Med J* 1965;2: 1327-1332.

10. Stewart A, Webb J, Hewitt D: A survey of childhood malignancies *Br Med J* 1958;1: 1495-1508.

11. Stewart A, Kneale GW: Radiation dose effects in relation to obstetric x-rays and childhood cancers. *Lancet* 1970;1: 1185-1188.

12. Mancuso TF, Stewart A, Kneale G: Radiation exposure of Hanford workers dying from cancer and other causes. *Health Phys* 1977;33: 369-384.

13. Kneale G, Stewart A, Mancuso TF: Reanalysis of data relating to the Hanford study of the cancer risks of radiation workers, in Late Biological Effects of Ionizing Radiation. Vienna, Vol 1. International Atomic Energy Agency, 1978;(pp) 386-412.

14. Sternglass EJ: Comments before the Committee on the Biological Effects of Ionizing Radiations, 1980.

15. Bross IDJ, Natarajan N: Genetic damage from diagnostic radiation. *JAMA* 1977;237: 2399-2401.

16. Bross IDJ, Ball M, Falen S: A dosage response curve for the 1 rad range: Adult risks from diagnostic radiation. *Am J Publ Health* 1979;69: 130-136.

17. Lyon JL, Klanber MR, Garnder JW, et al: Childhood leukemias associated with fallout from nuclear testing. *N Engl J Med* 1979;300: 397-402.

18. Court-Brown WM, Doll R, Hill AB: The incidence of leukemia following exposure to diagnostic radiation in utero. *Br Med J* 1960;2: 1539-1545.

19. Jablon S, Kato H: Childhood cancer in relation to prenatal exposure to atomic-bomb radiation. *Lancet* 1970;72: 1000-1003.

20. Gilbert ES, Marks S: An analysis of mortality of workers in a nuclear facility. *Radiat Res* 1979;79: 122-148.

21. Hatchison GB, MacMahon B, Jablon S, et al: Review of the report by Mancuso, Stewart and Kneale of radiation exposure of Hanford workers. *Health Phys* 1979;37: 207-220.

22. National Research Council, Advisory Committee on the Biological Effects of Ionizing Radiation: The Effects on Populations of Exposure to Low Levels of

Ionizing Radiations. Washington DC, National Academy of Sciences, 1980.

23. Oppenheim BE: Genetic damage from diagnostic radiation? *JAMA* 1979;242: 1390-1393.

24. Boice JD, Land CE: Adult leukemia following diagnostic x-rays? *Am J Pub Health* 1979;69: 137-145.

25. Land CE: The hazards of fallout or of epidemiologic research? *N Eng J Med* 1979;300: 431-432.

26. Archer VE: Geomagnetism, cancer, weather and cosmic radiation. *Health Phys* 1978;34: 237-247.

27. Frigerio NA, Stowe RS: Carcinogenic and genetic hazards from background radiation, in Biological and Environmental Effects of Low-Level Radiation. Vienna, International Atomic Energy Agency, 1976; pp 384-393.

28. Neel JV, Kato H, Schull WJ: Mortality in the children of atomic bomb survivors and controls. *Genetics* 1974;76: 311-326.

29. Selby PB: Genetic effects of low-level irradiation, in Fullerton GD, et al (eds) *Biological Risks of Medical Irradiations*. Medical Physics Monograph No. 5. American Association of Physicists in Medicine, 1980, p. 1-20. New York, American Institute of Physics, 1980;pp: 1-20.

30. Selby PB, Selby PR: Gamma-ray induced dominant mutations that cause skeletal abnormalities in mice. I. Plan, summary of results and discussion. *Mutat Res* 1977;43: 357-375.

6.

Radiation Measurements and Units of Radiation Quantity

Marc Edwards

A prerequisite to any study of biologic or epidemiologic effects of radiation is the ability to detect and quantify the various types of radiation in an accurate manner. Two distinct circumstances of radiation must be considered, namely those of external fields and those of internally deposited radionuclides. Furthermore, two distinct types of radiation descriptors need to be developed: those that correlate with the physical processes of energy deposition in matter and those that correlate with the ultimate biologic effects. Unlike the early period of investigations into radiation effects, it is our fortune not only to have solved a large portion of radiation problems, but also to have agreed on internationally accepted standards and definitions. Radiation dosimetry and radiation protection quantities and units are periodically reviewed and defined at the international level by the International Commission on Radiation Units and Measurements (ICRU) and by the International Commission on Radiological Protection (ICRP). In the United States, the National Bureau of Standards (NBS) and National Council on Radiation Protection and Measurements (NCRP) provide similar services. Most of this discussion comes from these sources.

At the outset it is well to recall the difference between a quantity and its unit. A "quantity" is loosely defined as a property or parameter of a substance the definition of which permits precise numerical measurement of the amount of that substance. Each quantity may have one or more "units" that define a standardized amount of that quantity such that measurements can be described in multiples of the unit. For instance, if, instead of health effects of low-level radiation, we were interested in the health effects of falling rock, a quantity of interest would be mass and its unit would be the kilogram. Various systems of units for physical quantities have been devised over the years, resulting in a variety of units for the same quantity. Quantities and units used in radiation dosimetry and protection have not escaped this proliferation of units. By recent agreement, the International System of SI units, which is based on the fundamental units of kilogram, meter, second, and ampere, is recommended for use in all technical and scientific communication. Hence, in this discussion both the older system of units, which is still in common use, and the newer SI units are presented.

Let us initially consider quantities and units applicable to external fields of radiation, closely following the treatment given in ICRU Report 33.[1] Historically the first radiation quantity to be defined precisely was "exposure." Although its definition has gone through several changes,[2] the current definition is now accepted as follows:

> The exposure X is the quotient of dQ by dm, where dQ is the absolute value of the total charge of the ions of one sign produced in air when all the electrons liberated by photons in a volume element of air having mass dm are completely stopped in air:

$$X = dQ/dm$$

The older special unit of exposure was the roentgen R, where

$$1R = 2.58 \times 10^{-4} \, \text{coul/kg air}$$

In the SI system, the roentgen has been abandoned, and no special unit of exposure has been defined other than its dimensions, expressed in coulombs per kilogram. The definition of the roentgen arose from an early ability and convenience of measuring ionization produced in air. Although its definition is an important step in quantifying radiation, it has several drawbacks. First, it is a measure of ionization produced in a particular medium, air, and does not translate readily to ionization in any other medium, such as soft tissue or bone. Second, it is defined only for one type of radiation, x- and γ-ray photons, and hence specifically does not apply to any other types of radiation, such as electrons, neutrons, and so forth. Finally, it turns out that the roentgen is not definable for high-energy photons, the upper limit being approximately 3 MeV.

The various inadequacies of the roentgen directed attention toward development of a quantity and unit that described the absorption of energy rather than the production of ionization, even though ionization continued to be the most prevalent way of measuring energy absorption. The quantity developed, now termed "absorbed dose," is defined as follows:

> The absorbed dose D is the quotient of $d\bar{\Sigma}$ by dm, where $d\bar{\Sigma}$ is the mean energy imparted by ionizing radiation to the matter in a volume element and dm is the mass of the matter in that volume element:

$$D = d\bar{\Sigma}/dm$$

The older special unit of absorbed dose was the rad, where

$$1 \text{ rad} = 10^{-2} \text{ J/kg}$$

In the system of SI units, absorbed dose is measured in grays (Gy), where

$$1 \text{ Gy} = 1 \text{ J/kg}$$

Note that 1 gray equals 100 rads. Absorbed dose may be defined in any medium, with any type of ionizing radiation and over any energy range. It should be noted, however, that absorbed dose is an average quantity; it does not describe the way in which the energy is imparted at a microscopic level or its temporal or spatial distribution.

Although exposure and, more often, absorbed dose are very important in quantifying a radiation field they do not constitute a complete description of radiation quantity. Absorbed dose by itself does not convey any information about the type of radiation, its spectral distribution, or its microdosimetric properties. The various quantities and units associated with these and other radiation field descriptors are thoroughly discussed by the ICRU.[1]

For radiation arising from the decay of radioactive nuclides, additional quantities and units are required. These descriptors will be necessary for the dosimetry of ingested or absorbed radioisotopes. The quantity of a radioactive nuclide may be defined by its activity as follows:

The activity A of an amount of radioactive nuclide in a particular energy state at a given time is the quotient of dN by dt, where dN is the expectation value of the number of spontaneous nuclear transitions from that energy state in the time interval dt:

$$A = dN/dt$$

The older special unit of activity was the curie (Ci), where

$$1 \text{ Ci} = 3.7 \times 10^{10} \text{ s}^{-1}$$

In the newer SI units systems, the curie has been dropped in favor of the becquerel (Bq), where

$$1 \text{ Bq} = \text{s}^{-1}$$

A convenient conversion from the older to the newer units system is as follows:

$$1 \text{ mCi} = 37 \text{ MBq}$$

Knowledge of the activity of a particular radioisotope is insufficient information to calculate the absorbed dose from that isotope. The additional information required is a complete description of the types of emitted radiations, their respective number of emissions per decay, and their respective energies. Using techniques outlined in ICRU Report 32[3] or in the earlier Medical Internal Radiation Dose (MIRD) Committee Reports, internal absorbed doses may be calculated. In its simplest formulation, the mean absorbed dose D to a target region is calculated by

$$D = A\Delta\Phi$$

where A is the number of nuclear transformations in a source region during the time interval of interest, Δ is the mean energy emitted per nuclear decay, and Φ is the fraction of the energy emitted by the source region and imparted to the target region per unit mass of the target region.

Although the formula appears simple, the amount of information necessary for its accurate application is considerable. The type and activity of the radionuclide administered, its physical half-life and decay data, the identity, location, mass, and shape of the target region, as well as the temporospatial distribution of activity in the source region must all be known. Partial compilation of these data, particularly as applied to medical isotopes, is given in ICRU 32 and MIRD reports, with much more extensive data for radiation protection applications available from the ICRP, as discussed below.

A knowledge of the quantities and units briefly reviewed above permits specification of the physical absorbed dose to any medium from external or internal radiation fields and sources. We should not expect, however, that a parameter as simple as average energy absorbed per unit mass will correlate uniquely with biologic effect. The number of cells damaged or killed by 1 gray of fast neutrons, 1 gray of ^{60}Co photons, 1 gray of soft x-rays, and 1 gray from a uniformly distributed α-emitting radioisotope will generally be quite different. This is because the quantity of absorbed dose fails to take into account several important physical phenomena and does not attempt even to consider mechanisms of biologic damage.

The most important physical phenomenon not described by absorbed dose is the manner in which energy is spatially deposited on a microscopic scale, often termed "microdosimetry." Owing to the random nature of radiation interactions, energy is deposited nonuniformly in small volumes. Thus, for volumes having dimensions typical of biologic targets, that is, microns or less, there is a high probability that no interaction will occur in that volume and hence no energy will be locally deposited. However, when an interaction does occur, the local energy deposition can be quite high.

Many quantities and units are associated with microdosimetry,[1] but time does not permit their complete discussion. One quantity that must be discussed, however, is linear energy transfer (LET). Charged particles, originating either as the primary radiation or secondarily from interactions of an uncharged primary radiation, lose energy attributable to collisions with electrons as they traverse a given material. As previously noted, this energy loss appears predominantly as the production of ionization. The rate of energy loss per unit path length is defined as LET. No special unit has been defined for this quantity, although dimensions of kiloelectron-volts per micron are typically used. It turns out that radiations that are themselves high-LET radiation, or that produce high-LET secondaries, result in microdosimetric distributions that have a significant probability of very large local energy deposition when an interaction occurs. For low-LET radiations, the probability of very large local energy deposition is much reduced. Neutrons and α particles are examples of high-LET radiations, while x-rays, γ-rays, and electrons are examples of low-LET radiations. Extensive radiobiologic research has shown that, for identical absorbed doses, high-LET radiations produce a greater biologic effect than do low-LET radiations. Hence, in developing a system of quantities and units for radiation effect correlation or radiation protection, LET must be taken into account.

Other physical phenomena can be important to biologic effects, but are not explicit in the definition of absorbed dose. For many biologic systems, the rate at which the dose is delivered can have a considerable effect on the amount of damage produced, particularly for low-LET radiations. This topic has been reviewed extensively by the NCRP.[4] In the case of internally absorbed alpha and beta emitters, the distribution of the radioisotope can have a significant effect on the homogeneity of dose deposition. This so-called "hot-particle" dosimetry has also received considerable attention.[5]

We are now in a position to discuss radiation quantities and units for radiation protection. It should be emphasized that radiation protection quantities and units, although precisely defined, must account for approximations and uncertainties inherent in operational radiation protection and safety programs. Hence they are designed to be conservative in the sense that they may overestimate the biologic effect. They are specifically not recommended for predicting or assessing the effects of high-level exposures.

The basic quantity of radiation protection,[6] called dose equivalent, is defined as follows:

The dose equivalent H is the product of D, Q, and N at the point of interest in tissue, where D is the absorbed dose, Q is the quality factor, and N is the product of all other modifying factors:

$$H = DQN$$

The older special unit of dose equivalent was the rem (the acronym for rad equivalent mammal), where

$$1 \text{ rem} = 10^{-2} \text{ J/kg}$$

The SI unit of dose equivalent is the sievert (Sv), where

$$1 \text{ Sv} = 1 \text{ J/kg}$$

Note that

$$1 \text{ Sv} = 100 \text{ rem}$$

The quality factor Q weights the absorbed dose for the biologic effectiveness of the charged particles producing the absorbed dose, and thus depends on the LET of the radiation. Although various graphs and conversion tables exist for determining quality factor from LET, they require a detailed knowledge of the LET distribution of the particular radiation field of interest. In the absence of such knowledge, the ICRP and other agencies have recommended a quality factor of 1 for x-rays, γ-rays, and electrons; a quality factor of 10 for neutrons and protons; and a quality factor of 20 for α-particles and other multiply-charged particles. The product of all other modifying factors N is currently assigned a value of 1 by the ICRU and ICRP, but is maintained in the definition for future use as knowledge about possible modifying factors becomes sufficient to justify some other value.

In the case of ingested or inhaled radionuclides we have previously noted the complexity inherent in absorbed dose calculations. For calculation of absorbed dose to a particular organ, not only must physical data concerning the type and amount of isotope be known, but also data must be collected on the chemical form of the isotope and its metabolism in the body. In addition, it is often difficult to detect and quantify internal isotopes, such that direct determination of organ doses is impossible. For these reasons, the control of internally deposited isotopes is focused on controlling their concentration in the environment. Fairly complex mathematical models that simulate the ingestion, inhalation, absorption, deposition, and retention kinetics of the various possible chemical forms of radionuclides are used to calculate the amount of radionuclide that results in a given level of organ dose. For some years, the quantities maximum permissible concentration (MPC) and maximum permissible body burden (MPBB) were used. The MPC was that concentration of radionuclide that, in continuous exposure to a standard man for a working lifetime of 50 years, would result in the worker containing the MPBB at the end of that period. The MPBB was estimated to deliver a dose-equivalent rate to the appropriate critical organ such that recommended limits on dose equivalent for any relevant stated period were not exceeded. The ICRP has recently recommended that the MPC and MPBB be discontinued.[7] This recommendation arose both from a perceived misapplication of MPC standards and the development of better internal dosimetry models. The new recommendations are based on the annual limit of intake (ALI), which is that activity of a radionuclide that taken alone would irradiate the reference man, considered as a whole rather than from the critical organ concept, to the limits set by the ICRP for each year of occupational exposure. This new quantity emphasizes the actual intake of radionuclides and recognizes that, depending on the circumstances, the older MPC values may be either exceeded or made more restrictive.

As can be seen from this brief review, the subject of radiation quantities and units, while generally well understood and defined, is undergoing constant refinement. For further information and updates, the reader is encouraged to review the references cited.

REFERENCES

1. International Commission on Radiation Units and Measurements: *Radiation Quantities and Units*. ICRU Report 33. Washington DC, ICRU, 1980.
2. Wyckoff HO: From "Quantity of Radiation" and "Dose" to "Exposure" and "Absorbed Dose" — An Historical Review, in *Quantitative Risk in Standards Setting*. Proceedings of the 16th Annual Meeting of the NCRP, Washington DC, 1980.
3. International Commission on Radiation Units and Measurements: *Methods of Assessment of Absorbed Dose in Clinical Use of Radionuclides*. ICRU Report 32. Washington DC, ICRU, 1979.
4. National Council on Radiation Protection and Measurements: *Influence of Dose and its Distribution in Time on Dose-Response Relationships for Low-LET Radiations*. NCRP Report 64. Washington DC, NCRP, 1980.
5. Richmond, CR: The importance of non-uniform dose-distribution in an organ. *Health Phys* 1975; 29:525–537.
6. International Commission on Radiation Units and Measurements: *Recommendations of the ICRP*. ICRP Publication 26. Elmsford, NY, Pergamon Press, 1977.
7. International Commission on Radiological Protection: *Limits for Intakes of Radionuclides by Workers*. ICRP Publication 30, Part 1. Elmsford, NY, Pergamon Press, 1979.

7.

Sources of Low-Level Radiation Exposure to the Public

E. Russell Ritenour

Radiation has always been part of the human environment. Cosmic rays emanating from the many stars and starlike objects in our galaxy (including the sun) and beyond have bathed the earth in radiation for billions of years. Similarly, radioactive materials have existed in the earth's crust and in the air since the earth was formed. These two sources constitute what is known as "the natural background" of radiation. When materials of "natural" origin, such as wood, brick, and marble, are used to construct shelters for humans, these materials irradiate the occupants of the shelters. Modern technology has resulted in many new sources of radiation. Various consumer products, atomic weapons fallout, weapons production, the nuclear fuel cycle, and medical radiology account for about as much exposure to the public each year as does the omnipresent "natural radiation."

This chapter examines both natural and artificial sources of radiation. The diversity of sources and some estimates of radiation dose are also discussed. But first, a word of caution. Some sources do not distribute radiation uniformly within the body. For instance, alpha emitters deposit their energy in small regions. If an alpha emitter is external to the body, there will be a high dose on the skin surface and virtually no dose to internal organs. If an alpha emitter has been inhaled or ingested, there may be a high dose to particular organs where the alpha emitter is concentrated, and no dose to the rest of the body. Therefore, it is as important to know the region of the body being irradiated as it is to know the value of the absorbed dose caused by a particular source. The terms "whole-body dose" and "dose to all internal organs" are used where possible to indicate the impact of radiation on the entire organism.

NATURAL RADIATION

The processes by which objects in the universe emit the high-energy particles known as cosmic rays are not completely understood. The composition of cosmic rays in our corner of the galaxy is, however, well known. Cosmic rays consist mostly of protons (approximately 90 percent), with the remainder being alpha particles, heavy nuclei, and electrons, all having extremely high energies. Only about 1/1,000 of the cosmic radiation striking the earth's atmosphere penetrates to the earth's surface. These high-energy particles interact with the nuclei of atoms in the atmosphere and in the earth to produce radioactive isotopes. Thus there are two components to human cosmic ray exposure. One is direct radiation from cosmic ray particles. The other is radiation from atoms whose radioactivity was created by interaction with the cosmic rays. Radiation from radioactivity induced by cosmic rays contributes an average dose of 28 mrem/year to residents of the United States. Direct exposure to cosmic rays contributes an additional 0.7 mrem.[1] In higher elevations such as in the Rocky Mountain region, there is less atmosphere to shield persons from cosmic rays, and the dose estimates are nearly doubled.

Many of the radioactive elements in and on the earth were not formed by interactions with cosmic rays. Rather, they were present when the earth was formed and continue to decay with half-lives of billions of years, forming additional radioactive isotopes in the process. This part of natural background is referred to as "terrestrial." Potassium-40 makes the largest single contribution to the terrestrial background. It comprises about 0.01 percent of all potassium found in the world, including the potassium in crystal rock, plants, and human muscle tissue. We receive an annual dose to all organs of approximately 19 mrem from the potassium-40 contained within our own tissues. We receive an additional 8 mrem from external sources of potassium-40, such as from other people, soil, and food. Many other elements make small contributions to bring the total average whole-body dose rate from all external and internal terrestrial sources in the United States to about 53 mrem/year.[1] The figure is twice as high in the Rocky Mountains because of the granite rocks containing thorium and uranium in relatively high concentrations. The world average terrestrial background is approximately the same as in the United States, but unusual soil composition results in a few high background areas, such as the coast of Brazil (500 mrem/year), granite rock areas of France (265 mrem/year), the Northern Nile Delta (350 mrem/year), and parts of India (1,300 mrem/year).[2]

ARTIFICIAL RADIATION

Some of the radiation exposure that is artificially made could actually be said to be "technologically enhanced" natural radiation. We bring natural radioactive sources closer to us by using standard building materials, such as wood, granite, and brick. The dose rate attributable to these materials varies considerably owing to differences in ventilation, room size, inner wall material, and other factors. It has been estimated that the average dose rate to occupants of masonry buildings is at least 13 mrem/year to the whole body, while the dose rate in wood frame buildings is less than 10 mrem/year.[3] These values may be greater in poorly ventilated areas because of an increased concentration of radioactive radon gas. This situation may occur in the basements of "energy-efficient" homes, as the flow of outside air is purposely restricted. A limited study of another technologically enhanced source, highway and road construction materials, has indicated an average annual population dose of 0.1 mrem.[4]

There are many sources of radiation exposure that would not exist in the absence of modern technology. One example is fallout injected into the atmosphere from aboveground atomic weapon detonations. Although this source has not received the publicity in the 1980s that it did in the 1950s and 1960s, it is still present. The absorbed dose rate for the U.S. population is about 5 mrem/year,[5] resulting from aboveground use of atomic weapons. This dose rate will continue into the next century because of the long-lived isotopes found in the fallout from atomic blasts. While this amount is relatively insignificant in regard to health effects, it is alarming to note that such a lasting contribution to background radiation levels was made, for the most part, between 1945 and 1963. During that time, the United States conducted 231 aboveground detonations, 224 of which occurred at the Nevada Test site.[6] China and France have continued to conduct atmospheric blasts even though the United States and Russia stopped this practice after the signing of the 1963 Limited Test Ban Treaty.

Various consumer products contribute small amounts of radiation. A partial list of these sources is given in Table 1. Perhaps the most interesting

TABLE 1. RADIATION FROM CONSUMER PRODUCTS

Product	Dose (mrem/year)	Portion of Body Considered
Luminous wristwatches	1–3	Gonads
Television sets	0.3–1	Gonads
Coal combustion	0.25–4.00	Lungs
Oil combustion	0.002–0.004	Lungs
Gas ranges	6–9	Lungs
Tobacco products	8,000	Lungs
Uranium in dental porcelain (dentures and crowns)	60,000	Superficial layers of tissue in contact with teeth
Eyeglasses	1,000–4,000	Germinal cells of the cornea
Smoke detectors	0.03–1.5	Whole body

Data from National Council on Radiation Protection and Measurements Report No. 56, pp 55–57, 1977.

item on the list is tobacco. There is evidence that tobacco smoke contains relatively high concentrations of the radioactive isotopes lead-210 and polonium-210, which emit alpha particles. It has been estimated that for a 1.5-pack-a-day cigarette smoker who inhales, small areas of the bronchial lining of the lungs may be subjected to as much as 8,000 mrem/year.[7] This amount is 80 times the absorbed dose contributed by inhaled radioactive materials occurring normally in the air. There is a growing awareness in the medical research community that internal irradiation of this sort may contribute to the carcinogenicity associated with cigarette smoking.[8] The large values shown in Table 1 for dental porcelain and eyeglasses do not constitute health hazards, because the dose is distributed over a few millionths of an inch in comparatively insensitive tissues. Considering all known radioactive consumer products, the National Council on Radiation Protection and Measurements has determined that their total contribution to dose to the whole body is < 5 mrem.

There are several hundred nuclear reactors in operation in the United States. More than half of these reactors are used as propulsion units for naval vessels, some of which are outside U.S. territory at any one time. The rest of the reactors are used for research, training, and power generation. About 72 operational power reactors are licensed in the United States.[9] Supporting these reactors are various mines, mills, processing plants, and spent fuel storage sites. The Environmental Protection Agency (EPA) has set a limit on the whole-body dose to the general population of 25 mrem/year resulting from all activities in the nuclear power industry.[10] Estimates from the EPA show that the actual yearly dose to the U.S. population is currently on the order of 1 mrem.[11]

Medical radiation makes the single largest contribution to artificial radiation exposure. Radiation unavoidably accompanies modalities such as roentgenography and nuclear medicine. Here the absorbed dose to the patient is kept as low as possible, commensurate with obtaining the necessary diagnostic information. Radiation is also used therapeutically. In this case the dose is designed to be as high as possible to a tumor, while as low as possible to surrounding normal tissue. Of course, there are fundamental differences between medical irradiation of a population and most of the other sources of radiation discussed in this article. First, medical irradiation is not ubiquitous. Some persons may experience medical exposure in a given year, while others may not. Second, the radiation is received voluntarily as a result of a benefit/risk decision process that should involve the referring physician, the radiologist, and the patient. Finally, the radiation received can be carefully documented even years after a procedure has been done, because modern radiology departments keep track of the positioning of each patient in relationship to the source of radiation and the technique factors (e.g., x-ray tube voltage, current, and time) used for a particular type of study. The dose values given below are no better than estimates because exposure techniques for medical studies vary somewhat for different patients in different facilities. But, given the specific circumstances, a medical physicist can make a reasonably accurate estimate for a particular patient.

Approximately 65 percent of the U.S. population is exposed to x-rays for medical purposes each year. More than 50 percent of those exposed undergo radiographic procedures, while the rest experience dental diagnosis, fluoroscopy, nuclear medicine, and radiation therapy. Therapeutic radiologic procedures result in high exposures to limited regions of the body for a very small segment of the population and are not discussed further in this chapter.

In contrast to environmental exposures, medical procedures usually result in localized exposures. For example, an arm may be the only area exposed to a direct beam of x-rays. To compare the health impact of various partial body procedures, the average dose to the total bone marrow of the body can be estimated.[12] In comparison with other organs of the body, the bone marrow is very sensitive to radiation. Therefore, the dose to the total body supply of marrow can be used as an index of biologic effect. In diagnostic radiology, the total marrow dose varies from a few millirems for single views of extremities and for dental studies, to several hundred millirems for barium enemas and upper abdominal series. Nuclear medicine studies typically result in doses of several hundred millirems to the marrow.[13] Because of medical uses of radiation for some members of the public, the average exposure to the bone marrow of all people in the United States resulting from medical radiographic procedures was estimated in 1970 to be 103 mrem[12] by the Bureau of Radiological Health of the Food and Drug Administration.

Table 2 summarizes the major sources of low-level radiation exposure to the public. About half of the exposure is from "natural" sources; the other half is related to modern technology. However, along with this technology has come the ability to calculate, estimate, and measure extremely small amounts

TABLE 2. MAJOR SOURCES OF LOW-LEVEL RADIATION EXPOSURE
TO THE PUBLIC

Source	Dose to Internal Organ (mrem/yr)
Cosmic rays and cosmic ray-produced radioactive elements	29
Radioactive elements in the body	27
Terrestrial	26
Medical	100
Buildings	10–13
Fallout	5
Other technologies	5

of radiation. For instance, the radioactive isotopes contained in the paper on which this book is printed are giving you an absorbed dose rate of approximately 0.0005 mrem/hr in the region of your eyes.[14] It is hoped that the ability to make such estimates will continue to help society place new technologic sources of radiation into proper perspective.

REFERENCES

1. Natural Background Radiation in the United States. *Recommendations on the National Council on Radiation and Measurements*. Washington, D.C., New York, Report No 45. 1975.
2. Low Level Effects Fact Book. Prepared by the Low Level Effects Subcommittee of the Society of Nuclear Medicine, January 1981.
3. Oakley DT: *Natural Radiation Exposure in the United States*. Report ORP/SID 72-1. Washington DC, U.S. Environmental Protection Agency, Office of Radiation Programs, 1972.
4. Radiation Exposure from Consumer Products and Miscellaneous Sources. *Recommendations of the National Council on Radiation Protection and Measurements*. Report No 56. 1977.
5. The Effects on Populations of Exposure to Low Levels of Ionizing Radiation. Committee on the Biological Effects of Ionizing Radiations. Washington DC, National Academy of Sciences, 1980, p 85.
6. The Forgotten Guinea Pigs. Report Prepared for the use of the Committee on Interstate and Foreign Commerce United States House of Representatives, Committee *Pring* 96-IFC53, 96th Congress, 2d Session, August 1980.
7. Little JB, et al: Distribution of polonium in pulmonary tissues of cigarette smokers. *N Engl J Med* 1965; 273:1343.
8. Winters TH, DiFranzia RJ; Radioactivity in cigarette smoke. *N Engl J Med* 1982; 306: 6.
9. IEEE Spectrum: *IEEE* 1979; 16(11) 49.
10. U.S. Environmental Protection Agency: 40 CFR 190: *Environmental Radiation Protection Requirements for Normal Operations of Activities in the Uranium Fuel Cycle*. Report EPA 520/4-76-016, vol I. Washington DC, US Environmental Protection Agency, 1976.
11. US Office of Radiation Programs: *Radiological Quality of the Environment in the United States*, 1977. Report EPA 520/1-77-009. Washington, DC: US Environmental Protection Agency, Office of Radiation Programs, 1977.
12. Shlein B, et al: The Mean Active Bone Marrow Dose to the Adult Population of the United States from Diagnostic Radiology. Publication (FDA) 77-8013, Rochville, Md, US Dept of HEW-FDA, Bureau of Radiological Health, 1977.
13. Fullerton GD, et al (eds): Biological Risks of Medical Irradiations. New York, American Institute of Physics, 1980.
14. Lalit BY, et al: Radioactivity content of books. *Health Phys* 1981; 40:731.

8.

Basic Concepts of Epidemiology

David A. Savitz

DEFINITION AND CONCEPTUAL APPROACH

Epidemiology can be defined simply as the science of the distribution and determinants of disease in human populations.[1] As a descriptive tool, epidemiology can aid health care service providers, for example, in allocation of resources. In its analytic capacity, the epidemiologic approach can help identify determinants of disease through the study of human populations.

Epidemiology is primarily an observational rather than experimental methodology, with corresponding strengths and limitations. Relative to other approaches for assessing disease etiology and impacts of potential health hazards, epidemiology has a rather unique role that is complementary to, but independent of, both basic biologic sciences and clinical medicine. Experimental biologic sciences such as toxicology and physiology provide critical information on biologic mechanisms of disease required for causal inference. Clinical medicine often serves as the warning system that provides etiologic clues to be pursued through systematic investigation. The advantage of the epidemiologic approach is its reliance on human field experience, that is, the real world. While laboratory experimentation is uniquely well suited to defining potential hazards, it can neither determine whether human populations have actually been affected nor quantify that effect. Building all the complexities of human behavior and external factors into a laboratory study or mathematical model is impossible. By studying the world as it exists, epidemiology examines the integrated, summarized product of the myriad factors influencing health.

The weakness of the epidemiologic approach, as well as its strength, lies with its home in the community. Indeed, the epidemiologist's mission is to extract from the tangle of the real world the meaningful determinants of health. The conceptual and statistical complexities of epidemiology are necessary because people and communities do not organize themselves into well-

47

defined experimental protocols. We have the task of finding the experiment underlying the community's health experience and of drawing the appropriate conclusions from that experiment.

MEASURES OF ASSOCIATION

The fundamental concern in most epidemiologic studies can be thought of as the association between some exposure and some health measure. Exposure should be viewed broadly to include age, sex, and genetic factors, as well as radiation, drugs, or dietary exposures. More specifically, the underlying question is whether exposed persons have a different risk of developing a disease than do nonexposed persons.

Data from Shore et al[2] serve as a useful illustration of the essence of epidemiologic reasoning. The study was designed to determine whether women treated with x-rays for acute postpartum mastitis experienced a subsequent elevated risk of breast cancer as a result of that x-ray exposure. Shore et al[2] studied 571 women who were treated with x-rays for acute postpartum mastitis at a clinic between 1940 and 1955. They were followed through 1972 to determine whether they developed breast cancer. Although several comparison groups were included, for the moment consider only the group of 993 women not treated with x-rays. Before a comparison of the breast cancer risks in the two groups can be made, the risk in each group must be quantified. The incidence rate used by Shore et al.[2] was defined as the number of new cases of the disease (in this case, breast cancer) per population at risk (i.e., all women who did not already have breast cancer) over a defined time interval. For example, among the 571 women treated with x-rays, 37 were identified as having developed breast cancer through 1972. Ignoring losses to follow-up and duration of follow-up, the incidence rate would be measured as 37/571 or 0.065, or 64.8 per 1,000, women over the time span of the study. Similarly, the control group of 993 women experienced 34 incident breast cancers, for a rate of 34.2 per 1,000.

The most obvious ways of comparing the two groups are through ratio and difference measures. The risk ratio is simply the incidence rate in the exposed group (64.8/1,000) divided by the rate in the nonexposed group (34.2/1,000), or 1.89. Women exposed to x-rays were nearly twice as likely to develop breast cancer as compared with women not exposed to x-rays. The risk difference is the incidence rate among the exposed subjects minus the incidence rate among nonexposed subjects: 64.8/1,000 − 34.2/1,000 = 30.6/1,000. This measure suggests that for every 1,000 women exposed to x-rays, an additional 30.6 cases of breast cancer will result.

In many situations, it is advantageous to measure risk as cases per person-time rather than cases per person in the study. Although it is conceptually easier to think of persons as the risk unit, this approach raises certain problems. Persons may be observed for different time intervals attributable to different entry and withdrawal times, their observation may cover different calendar times, and the postexposure durations may differ.[3]

Because radiation epidemiology is often concerned with cancer risks, which vary over calendar time and in relationship to the time of radiation exposure, most investigators consider person-time to be the risk unit. The disease risk measure used by Shore and associates (and generally employed in follow-up studies) is in the form of cases per person-years at risk (PYR). For example, if 10 women were followed for 20 years each (200 PYR) and two breast cancers were to develop, the observed rate would be 1.0 cancers per 100 PYR. In the Shore et al. study, 37 breast cancers were observed over 14,184 PYR among exposed women, producing a crude (i.e., unadjusted) rate of 2.61 per 1,000 PYR. The comparable rate in nonirradiated women was 1.35 per 1,000 PYR. Thus, the relative risk was 2.61/1,000 ÷ 1.35/1,000 = 1.93 and the risk difference 2.61/1,000 − 1.35/1,000 = 1.26/1,000 PYR.

While the above overview introduces the elementary principles of quantifying risk, the information provided to this point on the study by Shore et al. is inadequate to draw any conclusions. What if the age compositions of the irradiated and nonirradiated group were notably different? What if some of the women received radiation at an age when they were not very sensitive to radiation carcinogenesis? Variables other than the primary exposure and health outcome must be considered.

CONSIDERATION OF EXTRANEOUS VARIABLES: CONFOUNDING, EFFECT-MODIFICATION, AND RELATED ISSUES

The major complication in observational investigations is the presence of other risk factors. Radiation is clearly not the sole determinant of breast cancer nor is it fair to assume that radiation exposure exerts the same effect on risk for all persons.

Confounding

The first concern is with confounding, which is the mixing of the effect of interest with other effects. Age is an easily appreciated potential confounder. Suppose we wished to examine the effect of radiation on the development of prostate cancer. If the exposed persons were aged 50-70 while our non-exposed group was aged 10-30, the effect of radiation exposure would be mixed with the effect of age. The observed excess risk among the exposed would be attributable primarily to the age difference. Confounding can be more subtle when the discrepancy in the age distributions is smaller. Also, this mixing of effects can spuriously hide a true effect as well as create an illusory one. All major risk determinants must be addressed as potential confounders. Age adjustment is routinely applied, but there is nothing magic about age as a risk factor other than that it is often a very strong determinant. Adjustment for smoking in lung cancer comparisons and for hypertension in stroke comparisons is just as necessary.

Potential confounders can be addressed in a number of ways. One way is simply to restrict the sample to being homogeneous on the potential confounder. Race is related to breast cancer risk, so Shore et al. restricted both exposed and nonexposed groups to white women. Another method of control is matching, either individually or by group. A Shore et al. control subgroup consisted of the sisters of irradiated cases to control for familial predisposition to breast cancer by matching on genetic factors.

The most frequently employed method of control is through statistical adjustment. For example, age adjustment is applied to compare two populations with different age distributions through computing their risks as if their age distributions were the same. The adjusted rates estimate what would have occurred if the groups had the same age distribution. Shore et al. adjusted for age in this manner with person-years rather than with persons serving as the analytic units. Since breast cancer risk varies by age, differences in the age distribution of the PYR in exposed and nonexposed groups could distort the comparisons, that is, cause a mixing of age effects with radiation effects. Shore et al. weighted the age-specific rates in the exposed women according to the distribution of person-years in the control series, producing an age-adjusted breast cancer incidence rate of 2.85/1,000 PYR compared with the crude rate of 2.61. Often, the extent of confounding is quantified by the difference between crude and adjusted relative risks. In this instance the crude relative risk was $2.61/1.35 = 1.83$ and the adjusted relative risk was $2.85/1.35 = 2.11$, indicating that age distorted the results very litte.

Another technique frequently employed to adjust for confounding in epidemiologic studies is indirect adjustments to produce standardized morbidity or mortality ratios (SMRs). Instead of deriving rates for exposed and nonexposed groups, the observed rates in a group (usually the exposed) are compared with what would be expected had their risks been equal to those in some reference (usually nonexposed) population. The expected number is standardized by calculating the number one would have observed if the study group had had the risk level of the reference group within each age group.

The ratio of the observed to the expected number of cases (the SMR) is intended to approximate the adjusted relative risk. Shore et al. employed age and calender-year specific incidence data from the New York State Cancer Registry in upstate New York to derive an expected number of breast cancer cases to be compared to the observed numbers. While 37 such cancers were observed in irradiated women, only 11.3 were expected had the women experienced the rates observed for women in upstate New York in each age interval and calendar period. The SMR, the observed number divided by the expected number, is 37/11.3 or 3.27 (sometimes expressed as a percent or 327). The control series had an SMR of 1.62 or 62 percent above the expected value.

Effect-Modification

Interaction or effect-modification occurs when the exposure-disease relationship itself differs as a function of some third variable or set of variables.[4] For example, it is often postulated that radiosensitivity varies in relation to age, with exposures at younger ages conferring greater cancer risk than equivalent exposures at later ages. In statistical terms, an exposure by age interaction is postulated.

Shore and co-workers addressed this question by calculating the relative risk separately for women first irradiated between ages 15-29 and women first irradiated at age 30 or older. The age-adjusted relative risk estimates were 2.2 for both groups, indicating an absence of effect-modification. A unit dose of radiation caused a constant proportionate increase in cancer risk regardless of age. Another type of effect-modification concerns the possibility that pre- and postmenopausal breast cancer might show differential radiosensitivity. To examine this, the relative risk for ages 25-49 (RR = 2.0) and ages 50-85 (RR = 2.5) were calculated showing little if any interaction.

Latency

The concept of latency, addressed thoroughly by Rothman,[5] is essential to the proper interpretation of epidemiologic research on the effects of radiation. In simplistic terms, some exposures are known to manifest their impact only after some substantial time interval has elapsed. Since radiation-induced cancers do not appear until some years after exposure, brief periods of follow-up after an exposure are inadequate to determine whether excess cancer risk has occurred.

Shore et al. were concerned that the duration of follow-up (interval since entry) might act to distort the results. It is generally agreed that cancer risk rises some time after irradiation, that is, a latency period occurs. If the study fails to recognize this, the observed effect may be diluted. For example, a 5-year observation after exposure to radiation in rather high doses would probably show no change in lung cancer risk. The basic assumption in a person-years analysis is that one person followed x years is the same as x people followed 1 year. Under the conditions described above, 1 year of observation during the latency is quite different than 1 year while the risk is manifested. Shore et al. observed a relative risk of 1.0 for follow-up years 0-9,

1.5 for years 10–19, and 3.6 for years 20–34. Clearly, the relative risk of radiation exposure did not fully develop until after 10 years of observation.

Dose Response

Radiation is universally acknowledged as a carcinogen. The more controversial aspect of this phenomenon is the nature of the dose–response function.[6] Causal inference is strengthened when such a relationship can be demonstrated.[7] Furthermore, regulatory agencies must set exposure limits on the basis of the shape of that dose–response curve. Most of the current discussion of this issue[6] is focused on the appropriate models for extrapolating to low doses, since (1) the relationship at high doses is rather well understood, and (2) epidemiologic studies are unlikely to provide precise empirical estimates in the very low-dose range.[8]

Shore et al. examined this issue by dividing the women who received radiation exposure into five groups: 40–149, 150–249, 250–349, 350–449, and 450–1,200 rad. Compared with controls who received no radiation, the relative risks across the intervals (in ascending order) were 1.5, 2.3, 2.9, 3.1, and 2.2. In spite of some inconsistency, a pattern of increasing risk with increasing dose can be observed.

Relative Risk and Risk Difference

The decision of calculating risk versus risk difference relates to the question of whether radiation multiplies or adds to the baseline risk. If, for example, radiation were to double the risk for all age groups, the risk difference would rise across the age scale, since background risk increases with age (Fig. 1). Conversely, if radiation added a constant excess number of cases at all ages, it

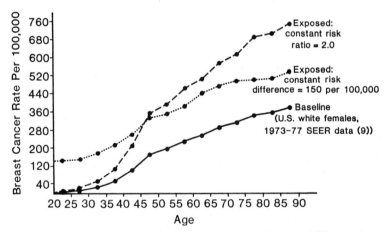

Figure 1. Constant proportional (ratio) versus constant absolute (difference) excess in radiation–induced breast cancer risk.

would produce dramatic relative risks at early ages (low background risk) declining sharply with advancing age (high background risk) (Fig. 1.) The data from Shore et al. are not definitive, but it appears that relative risk is constant across age (RR = 2.0 for ages 25–49 and RR = 2.5 for ages 50–85). The risk difference thus rose across the age groups, from 6.5/10^6 PYR/rad in 25–49-year-olds to 11.5/10^6 PYR/rad in 50–85-year-olds.

STUDY DESIGN

Two commonly used strategies for assessing the association between long-term exposures and chronic diseases are case-control (retrospective) and cohort (prospective) studies. These study designs are named for the sampling method employed. Case-control studies compare the exposure histories of people with a particular health problem (cases) with those of a reference group (controls). Cohort or prospective studies sample based on exposure or other potential etiologic factors and assess disease rates as the outcome measures.

Two clear illustrations of these methods in the study of radiation exposure and leukemia are by Gibson et al.[10] and Boice and Hutchison.[11] In the Tri-State Leukemia Study of Gibson et al., 1,414 adult leukemia cases and 1,370 adult controls were selected in upstate New York, Minneapolis, and Baltimore. Each of the cases and controls was interviewed to assess his or her history of exposure to diagnostic x-rays. The relative excess of radiation exposure reported by cases as compared to controls indicates an association. Usually the odds ratio (the ratio of the odds of exposure in controls to the odds of exposure in cases) is used as the estimate of relative risk. In the Gibson et al. study of acute and chronic myeloid leukemia, the proportion of male cases with high frequencies of diagnostic x-ray exposure was excessive compared with that of the controls, indicating an association.

The prospective design employed by Shore et al.[2] and by Boice and Hutchison[11] is, in many respects, easier to understand, since it proceeds from purported cause to effect. Boice and Hutchison identified 28,490 women treated with radiation for cervical cancer and 2,729 women with cervical cancer but not treated with radiation. Both groups' risks of developing leukemia were analyzed, with the rationale that excessive leukemia in radiation-exposed as compared with nonexposed women would be suggestive of a causal association between radiation exposure and subsequent leukemia. In the study by Boice and Hutchison, no association was observed.

Mausner and Bahn[1] provide a succinct summary of the strengths and weaknesses of these two study designs. Case-control studies have lower costs, require fewer subjects (assuming the disease is rarer than the exposure of interest), and produce results more quickly than cohort studies. It is the method of choice in studying rare diseases. The disadvantages of case-control studies include the possibility of biased recall of exposures, unavailability of desired information, inherent controversy in control group selection, and inability to directly produce absolute risk estimates (only relative risk is directly estimable). Cohort studies have several advantages: exposure classification is inherently unbiased because disease status is not yet known at the time of selection, incidence rates can be derived directly, and many health end points can be assessed within the same study. The disadvantages are the high cost associated with the need for lengthy follow-up and a large number of study subjects, as well as the possibility of bias in ascertainment of disease.

One form of prospective study, known as the historical prospective or retrospective cohort study design, avoids many of these problems. The design is simply a cohort study occurring over a previous time period. For example, instead of identifying a cohort receiving radiation exposure in 1982 and observing them for cancer through the year 2020, it is more efficient to identify a cohort exposed to radiation in 1940 and see what their health experience has been through 1980. These designs are conceptually identical but differ tremendously in their practicality. Both Shore et al.[2] and Boice and Hutchison[11] illustrate this method.

Which study design is optimal depends on the particulars under study. In the example of radiation and cancer, case-control studies can be argued for primarily because cancer is a rare disease and the latency period may be very long. Prospective studies have the noteworthy advantage of not relying on subjective memories of radiation exposures. The historical prospective design has emerged, with good reason, as the optimal approach to the identification of the health effects of radiation on human populations; it combines the accurate exposure assessment of a cohort design with the feasibility of a case-control design.

CAUSAL INFERENCE

The ultimate purpose for which epidemiologic data are gathered is to identify and characterize causal associations. At times, scientists attempt to restrict the notion of "cause" to a level of purity that epidemiologic results can never reach, for example, quibbling over whether cigarette smoking has been proved as a cause of lung cancer. The mainstream of epidemiologic thinking recognizes that the inference of causality lies on a continuum. As the evidence accumulates and is corroborated, scientists are swayed toward the belief that an etiologic association is present.

MacMahon and Pugh,[12] and more recently Schlesselman,[13] have discussed considerations (not rules) in distinguishing causal from noncausal associations. First, the putative cause must precede the health effect. Second, the association should be observed consistently under diverse study conditions. For instance, excess cancers have been observed following radiation from atomic bombs, medical treatments, and uranium mining. Third, a strong association, of course, is more supportive of causality than a weak association, although weak causes may still be real causes.[14] Fourth, a dose-response gradient supports a causal relationship.

Finally, the epidemiologic association should be consistent with existing knowledge, but support from the biologic sciences or aggregate population data (e.g., secular trends or international comparisons) is not essential in making causal inferences. Epidemiologists may be the first to discover a cause followed by laboratory science support.

Epidemiologists challenge assertions of causality by trying to discredit the research findings with noncausal explanations. Examination of spurious patterns of disease reporting (e.g., diagnostic fashions, accuracy) or exposure reporting (e.g., faulty memory in self-report) helps in the assessment of the value of the study. Such criticism is extremely useful for identifying where the major weaknesses lie and pointing toward the methodologic refinements needed in the next study. The epidemiologist's self-criticizing is sometimes misinterpreted as a flaw in the methodology. On the contrary, recognition of the weaknesses of each given study improves the quality of the causal inferences derived from a set of imperfect investigations.

Evaluation of the major chronic diseases and environmental health risks requires a clear recognition of multifactorial etiology. Simply put, there is rarely a single necessary or sufficient cause.[14] One can acquire leukemia without any anthropogenic radiation exposure, and one can receive substantial doses of radiation without acquiring leukemia. In the realm of radiation carcinogenesis, the causal link is universally accepted. The questions revolve around quantification of that risk, the timing of exposure and risk development, and the identification of radiosensitive subsets of persons and cancers.

REFERENCES

1. Mausner JS, Bahn AK: *Epidemiology: An Introductory Text*. Philadelphia, WB Saunders, 1974.
2. Shore RE, Hempelmann LH, Kowaluk E, et al: Breast neoplasms in women treated with x-rays for postpartum mastitis. *J Natl Cancer Inst* 1977;59: 813–822.
3. Morgenstern H, Kleinbaum DG, Kupper LL: Measures of disease incidence used in epidemiologic research. *Int J Epidemiol* 1980;9: 97–104.
4. Miettinen OS: Confounding and effect-modification. *Am J Epidemiol* 1974;100: 350–353.
5. Rothman KJ: Induction and latent periods. *Am J Epidemiol* 1981;114: 253–259.
6. Radford EP: Human health effects of low doses of ionizing radiation: The BEIR III controversy. *Radiat Res* 1980;84: 369–384.

7. Weiss NS: Inferring causal relationships: Elaboration of the criterion of "dose-response." *Am J Epidemiol* 1981;113: 487-490.

8. Land, CE: Estimating cancer risks from low doses of ionizing radiation. *Science* 1980;209: 1197-1203.

9. Young JL Jr, Percy CL, Asire AJ: *Surveillance, Epidemiology, and End Results: Incidence and Mortality Data, 1973-77.* U.S. DHHS Publ No (NIH) 81-2330. Washington DC, US GPO, 1981.

10. Gibson R, Graham S, Lilienfeld A, et al: Irradiation in the epidemiology of leukemia among adults. *J Natl Cancer Inst* 1972;48:301-311.

11. Boice JD, Hutchison GB: Leukemia in women following radiotherapy for cervical cancer: Ten-year follow-up of an international study. *J Natl Cancer Inst* 1980;65: 115-129.

12. MacMahon B, Pugh TF: *Epidemiology: Principles and Methods.* Boston, Little, Brown, 1970.

13. Schlesselman JJ: *Case-Control Studies. Design, Conduct, Analysis.* New York, Oxford, 1982.

14. Rothman KJ: Causes. *Am J Epidemiol* 1976;104:587-592.

9.

Review of Epidemiologic Studies of Hanford Workers: Cancer Risk and Low-Level Radiation

David A. Savitz

OVERVIEW

The extensive knowledge that has accumulated regarding long-term health effects of radiation is based on experiences of humans at relatively high doses. The most informative and well-known populations that have provided the current estimates of radiation's carcinogenicity are the Japanese atomic bomb victims and patients receiving therapeutic radiation for diseases such as ankylosing spondylitis.[1] Unfortunately, in spite of improved understanding of radiation biology and the thorough investigation of carcinogenic mechanisms, extrapolation of these risk estimates to much lower doses is fraught with uncertainty. Radford[2] has reviewed the controversy within a committee of informed radiation scientists on this issue, giving some indication of the confusion engendered among less-informed parties. In one sense, human experience provides the only empirical basis for determining human risks at low-dose levels. Unfortunately, as the focus moves to increasingly lower dose levels, the ability to characterize the shape of the dose–response curve accurately diminishes[3]; that is, lower doses imply a less pronounced excess of cancer occurrence, leading to lower precision in the dose–effect estimate.

The traditional (presumably conservative) approach to estimating the low-dose effects of radiation is linear extrapolation from the higher dose levels.[1] In the case of cancer induction, for example, if x rem produces an extra y cancers per person-years, $x/2$ rem is predicted to produce an extra $y/2$ cancers, and so on, down to 0 rem dose producing 0 extra cancers. This functional form has been debated extensively with arguments on both sides, i.e., that it underestimates or overestimates the true risk. Nonetheless, convincing data to resolve this debate have not yet emerged.

Gilbert and Marks[4] have noted that only if the current risk estimates are extremely understated is it likely that data on workers such as those at Hanford could clarify the nature of the radiation–cancer association. The initial and continuing interest in studying workers employed at the Hanford facility is to examine empirically the cancer risk associated with exposure to low-level radiation. If one envisions the functional relationship between radiation dose and cancer risk graphically, this study can be seen as having been designed to fill in a point on the lower portion of the dose–response curve and to address empirically the assumption of linear risk down to 0 dose.

The data set consists of records for all employees at the Hanford Works in Richland, Washington. The plant has been engaged in a variety of radiation-related activities, including plutonium manufacture, separation, and purification, as well as research in nuclear energy.[4] Each worker hired at the plant was monitored annually for whole-body external radiation exposure. Cause-specific mortality was noted for each deceased employee as obtained through records of the Social Security Administration and death certificates. For each person hired, the work history (dates of entering and leaving each position), annual measures of external and internal radiation, sex, date of birth, date of hire, and date and cause of death were noted.[5] Note that the only potential confounders available for consideration were sex, age, and calendar year. The level of precision in the exposure estimates relative to those commonly available in epidemiologic studies is quite impressive.

The fundamental research questions asked of the data must be kept firmly in mind in spite of the confusing technical details and unprecedented controversy. The first issue is simply whether radiation exposure in the dose ranges experienced by Hanford workers is associated with cancer risk. The additional concern is with refinements of that relationship: (1) Is there a dose–effect gradient and, if there is, what is its shape? (2) What is the time course of development and cessation of any increased risk? (3) Is there differential sensitivity to radiation doses incurred at different ages? (4) How does the risk differ across cancer types? (5) Can the observed cancer patterns be explained by other risk factors (confounders)?

The basic epidemiologic principles outlined in Chapter 8 are applicable to this research area and, in fact, are the best method of attempting to resolve the controversies. At the same time, the bounds of epidemiologic analysis and interpretation must be appreciated. Some questions, although of major political and public health significance, simply cannot be resolved with the tools of epidemiology. Issues such as the acceptability of certain observed risks or what decisions to make in the face of uncertainty are not within the domain of epidemiologic reasoning.

Perhaps the most important epidemiologic principle to be appreciated is the fallibility of any single observational study. Chance events and unmeasured or inadequately controlled confounders contribute to the outcome of any investigation. The results of a study contribute to a body of knowledge with a weight proportional to the overall quality of the research. The quality of that research and the degree of confidence one should place in the various (contradictory) results are addressed in this discussion.

REVIEW OF MAJOR STUDIES

Mancuso et al.[5]

The study that initiated the intense interest in the Hanford workers was that reported by Mancuso et al.[5] On the basis of mortality data over the period 1944–1972, the cumulative radiation dose received by cancer cases was compared with the doses received by persons dying from other causes.

Survivors were excluded in an attempt to adjust for the fact that survivors who worked for longer periods had notably higher radiation doses. The exposure measure was alternately defined as "percent exposed," "mean cumulative dose for exposed workers," and "mean cumulative dose for all workers." The last definition is the most comprehensive exposure measure for this group and serves as the primary exposure variable in the present review.

The results of the simple comparisons indicated higher cumulative mean doses (CMD) for all cancers, lung cancers, and colon cancers, in comparison with the CMD for persons dying from other causes. The cancer/noncancer comparison was further explored in reference to the calendar year of the exposure, the employment year (time since hire), predeath year, exposure age, and age at death. Each of these factors was investigated through determination of the percentage of exposed workers in each period or age and the average dose to exposed workers, as well as through assessment of how many of the years demonstrated higher CMDs for cancer victims. All are rather weak measures of exposure compared with the more direct measure of dose in rems.

Tests for interaction between radiation exposure and the other variables were conducted with rather unusual techniques including sign tests and a series of Student's t-tests across the variable posited to interact with radiation exposure. No interaction was apparent for calendar year or employment year, but there were interactions with predeath year and age of exposure. Exposure 8–20 years predeath showed a more pronounced excess in cancer cases, and exposures after age 35 showed a stronger association with cancer/noncancer status. Stratification by age at death indicated that the proportion of deaths due to cancer rose across a gradient of increasing CMD only for those in the 50–59 and 70+ age strata.

The efforts of Mancuso et al. to determine a doubling dose follow from the unsupported assumption that radiation was causally related to cancer in these workers, which is the focus of this review. Hutchison et al.[14] reviewed in some detail their rationale and methods for calculation of a doubling dose and found them to be deficient. Similarly, the effort to determine maximally sensitive predeath years and ages was simply a selection of the most impressive times to compare CMDs in cancer cases and the (other causes of death) controls. Predeath intervals of maximum contrast were 12 years for total cancers, 11 years for reticuloendothelial system cancers, 9 years for bone marrow cancer, less than 1 year for pancreatic cancer, and 14 years for lung cancer.

Kneale et al.[6]

Kneale et al.[6] reanalyzed the same data set with four major modifications, in which (1) deaths through 1977 were included; (2) stratification was carried out simultaneously on sex, age at death, internal radiation, and exposure period; (3) cancer aggregates based on ICRP definitions of radiosensitivity were analyzed; and (4) dose intervals and their corresponding odds ratios were examined. Again, the basic comparison was of CMD in persons dying from cancer (or a subset of cancers) compared with persons dying from other causes.

Simultaneous stratification of the potential confounders noted above (sex, age at death, year of death, internal radiation, exposure period) suggested that a small risk gradient in relationship to radiation exposure was present. The adjusted odds ratios (with a reference of 1.00 in those with <80 mrad) was 0.86 for the 80-310-mrad interval, 1.08-1.15 for 320-5110 mrad, and 1.26 above 5110 mrad. Classification of cancer radiosensitivity by the ICRP method suggested higher doses in those dying from the most radiosensitive cancers, consistent with the expectation if the association were causal. Analysis by predeath interval, however, suggested that the exposure differentials occurred exclusively in the 15-year period before death, contrary to most assumptions about latency periods for induction of cancer.

The basic changes in results from the earlier study were a revision in the magnitude of the estimated risk and a reduced list of "sensitive" cancers that included bone marrow, lung, and colon-stomach-pancreas. In addition, the introduction of an external classification of sensitive cancers indicated a higher CMD for radiosensitive cancers than for other cancers.

Gilbert and Marks[4]

A completely independent analysis of cancer mortality risks was undertaken by Gilbert and Marks.[4] In this analysis a more traditional occupational mortality analysis was employed of the 12,679 monitored white male employees employed at least 2 years. The Gilbert and Marks analysis considered survivors as well as deceased employees in analyzing the risks associated with radiation exposure. The vital status was ascertained through April 1, 1974, with a May 1, 1977 update leaving the results unchanged.[7] Preliminary analysis of cumulative radiation doses indicated a highly skewed distribution with <15% receiving doses over 1 rem/year and <1% receiving doses over 4 rem/year. Dose was concentrated in craftsmen and operators and closely correlated with calendar year and with continued employment.

Hanford workers were compared with the U.S. population (adjusted for age and calendar year), but emphasis was placed on internal comparisons by level of radiation dose received (0-2, 2-5, 5-15, and 15 + rem) with simultaneous consideration of age, calendar year, occupation, and employment status. Since radiation exposures temporally close to the time of death are presumably unrelated to that death (i.e., there is some latency period), the analyses were conducted with both 2- and 10-year lags in the dose accumulation.

Comparisons with the U.S. population revealed a standardized mortality ratio (SMR) of 0.88 among those employed <2 years and an SMR of 0.85 for those employed 2 + years, consistent with the "healthy worker effect." This indicates that the cancer deaths were only 88 percent of what would have been predicted based on the total U.S. white male population. The only elevated risks for specific cancer sites were for employees of <2 years who had an SMR for pancreatic cancer of 1.30 and for "residual" cancers of 1.34, but these excesses were attributable to deaths among nonexposed workers. The comparisons of cancer risk by exposure status indicated no trend of increasing risk with increasing exposures for total cancers or for any cancer sites except pancreas and multiple myeloma. Both patterns were attributable to three cases in the highest exposure interval compared to 0.5 (pancreas) and 1.0 (multiple myeloma) expected cases. The effect of eliminating exposures in the most recent 10 years before death was to eliminate the trend for pancreatic cancer. Otherwise, the results were generally insensitive to adjustment for employment status, occupation, 2-year predeath dose lag, hire year, length of employment, and subdivision of the lowest exposure interval.

Sanders[8]

Sanders[8] analyzed certain facets of the Hanford employee population pertinent to the assessment of a link between radiation exposure and cancer mortality. In an analysis restricted to exposed employees, he noted that the radiation dose increased substantially with calendar time while the proportion of deaths due to cancer over that interval (1944-1972) did not increase concurrently. Furthermore, stratification by year of death indicated that the cancer victims had not, in the majority of years, accumulated higher doses than other deceased persons.

Additional comparisons of cancer deaths with the total cohort showed a reverse gradient: cancer victims had lower cumulative exposures than the aggregate of other employees. Consideration of production workers hired in 1944–1945 or restriction to long-term employees did not alter these negative findings.

Gofman[9]

Gofman[9] chose to ask the question of whether radiation doses were related to cancer risk by contrasting persons with <10-rad and >10-rad of exposure. He attempted to allow for a latency period in cancer induction by restricting his study to workers who survived more than 15 years after hire. Basically the method adopted was a form of proportionate mortality analysis in which the proportion of deaths due to cancers was compared in the two dose groups (<10 versus 10 + rad). Several potentially confounding variables were considered, and differences in age at hire were addressed with a regression adjustment made by adding a derived number of noncancer cases to the high-dose group.

The result of the comparison of the proportion of cancer deaths in high- and low-dose groups was a marginally significant relative cancer excess in the high exposure group (38 vs. 25 percent). The possibility of a chemical rather than radiological cause was pursued through restriction of the study groups to long-term (11 or more years) employees under the assumption that any cumulative chemical effect would be manifest among long-duration employees. This adjustment for duration of employment increased rather than decreased the difference in proportions in the two exposure groups. Breakdown of deceased workers into the two dose groups <5 rad and 5–10 rad produced no difference in the proportion of deaths due to cancer, suggesting that any detectable carcinogenic effects were restricted to persons with a dose of ⩾10 rad.

Gofman examined specific cancer sites using a form of proportionate cancer mortality analysis, asking whether the proportion of persons with cancer of particular sites exceeding 10 rad was greater than expected on the basis of the total cancer experience. An array of the various cancers demonstrated essentially no pattern of sensitive cancer sites, though statistical testing of selected sites such as multiple myeloma would suggest increased radiosensitivity. Reanalysis by the ICRP classification of degree of radiosensitivity failed to indicate a gradient of increasing proportions of cases with high doses in relationship to the radiosensitivity of the cancer.

Kneale et al.[10]

The third analysis of the Hanford data by the original authors [10] provided three major modifications: (1) use of the Cox regression model for life tables as the statistical approach; (2) detailed examination of radiosensitive and other cancers as a clear dichotomy; and (3) use of internal radiation monitoring levels as a form of adjustment for what was considered a selection factor. It was argued that the most hazardous jobs involved extreme selection of healthy workers at hire and that control for the index of hazard in the form of internal radiation monitoring and whether radionuclides were, in fact, detected adjusts for this selection. The statistical methodology can be viewed as a regression model predicting survival or, for particular causes of mortality, failure to incur the fatal disease of interest.

Preliminary results predicting total mortality showed a strong protective effect of radiation exposure, which Kneale and associates viewed as "contrary to the facts." Introduction of various sorts of adjustments produced considerable changes in the results; that is, adjustment for sex, year of hire, and "job hazard index" gave a statistically significant coefficient indicating a positive relationship for radiosensitive cancers. Further analyses of proportionate mortality were carried out after eliminating deaths due to accidents and myocardial infarction and adjusting for place of death. This eliminated the previously observed apparent protective effect of radiation on total cancers while radiosensitive cancers still showed an association with cumulative radiation dose.

Darby and Reissland[11]

Interestingly, the most recently reported analysis of these data by Darby and Reissland[11] is probably the most thorough and conventional in terms of methods in occupational epidemiology and probably the most readily interpreted. All white employees who worked at Hanford for 2+ years were considered, with mortality ascertained through April 1, 1974. Person-years at risk were stratified by age, calendar year, time since hire, and radiation dose (discounting the most recent 2 years). Additional tests discounting the past 10 years of dose and counting only the dose in the preceding 2-10-year interval were performed as well. A test for trend of increasing risk with increasing dose served as the primary method of analysis (internal comparisons) supplemented with a traditional SMR analysis with expected rates based upon the U.S. white male population.

Overall mortality tended to decrease with increasing (recent) dose. In spite of testing 64 different cause of death groupings with three different dose lags (2, 10, and 2-10 only), few suggestions of a radiation effect were detected. Nonlymphatic leukemia and hematopoietic cancers were associated with dose as of >10 years ago, attributable exclusively to the strongly positive findings for multiple myeloma. For this disease, three cases above a dose of 5 rem were observed, while only 0.28 were expected. A similar pattern appeared for renal and pancreatic cancers, with the effect primarily due to doses more than 10 years ago for renal cancer and very recent doses for pancreatic cancer.

SMRs based on U.S. rates showed the usual selectively low mortality that diminished over the years after hire. The SMR for total cancers was 0.80, with only multiple myeloma showing an excess (SMR = 1.14) based on 0.9 excess cases. Based on a 10-year dose lag, there was a 10-fold excess of multiple myeloma among persons with >5 rem, and small excess for pancreatic cancer (SMR = 1.54) and renal cancer (SMR = 1.67) in the same dose group. Given the small number of high-dose kidney cancers (only 1) and the fact that pancreatic cancer is really unlikely to be induced by a very recent dose, Darby and Reissland concluded that only multiple myeloma showed firm evidence of an association with radiation dose.

General Accounting Office[12]

As part of a comprehensive review of cancer risks and low-level radiation, the GAO[12] reviewed the study by Mancuso et al.[5] performing their own analyses as an outgrowth of that critique. The data analyzed included all white male workers employed at Hanford for 2 or more years, with deaths ascertained through 1978. The GAO analysis was motivated specifically by a desire to determine why the earlier results have been discrepant. Beginning with the simplest model, which was very similar to that of Mancuso et al.,[5] this investigative group introduced refinements sequentially, up to an analysis very similar to the Cox regression of Kneale et al.[10] or the life-table approaches of Gilbert and Marks[4] and Darby and Reissland.[11]

A simple regression of cumulative radiation dose on the presence or absence of a specific cause of death (among deceased workers) essentially replicated the work of Mancuso et al.[4] Unadjusted estimates suggested slightly higher doses for all cancers displaying a more marked elevation for radiosensitive cancer sites. Among specific cancer sites, pancreas and multiple myeloma showed statistically significant elevations.

The second analysis considered the time at risk for the deceased workers and adjusted for year of hire, age at hire, and calendar period at risk. Dose was lagged by 4 years. Results with these adjustments indicated a significant association for radiosensitive cancers as well as multiple myeloma and pancreatic cancer. All cancers and solid tumors appeared to be independent of the level of radiation exposure with these adjustments.

A model of relative risk in relationship to radiation exposure was developed to test multiplicative effects of radiation with other risks as distinct from the additive assumption in the linear regression models discussed above. Results are quite similar to all the others; there is no association with total cancers, a marginal association with radiosensitive cancers, and a statistically significant association with multiple myeloma and pancreatic cancer.

Several other analyses reported in the appendix to the GAO report vary such factors as the inclusion of survivors and the consideration of different potential confounders. It is interesting that the above conclusions are insensitive to the analytic methods, that is, no association between radiation and total cancers, a borderline association with radiosensitive cancers, and a consistent association with pancreatic cancer and multiple myeloma attributable to a few highly exposed decedents.

METHODS

A review of the eight approaches demonstrates that the same question—Is radiation exposure related to cancer risk in Hanford workers?—can be addressed in many different ways. It should also be appreciated that there is no one best approach to answering such questions. There are, however, epidemiologic principles through which these studies can be evaluated with an overall indication of the validity of the results and conclusions.

There is relatively little controversy about how to measure exposure, since personal dosimeter readings were available for each year. The quality of such information relative to the exposure information employed in most occupational health studies is quite impressive, although it is not possible to address nonoccupational radiation exposure adequately, even though they are of the same order as the occupational doses.[13] In addition, it is commonly thought that workers subvert the monitoring program to avoid the threatened layoffs if exposures exceed the limit. Both factors tend to underestimate the true total dose, biasing the estimated health risks per unit dose downward.

An important initial question is how to treat dose statistically, that is, as a continuous variable or in discrete categories. If the dose–response function for radiation is linear, then dose treated as a continuous variable has the most statistical power to detect effects on cancer risk.[6] If, however, there is any nonlinearity over the dose range observed in the form of a threshold as implied by Gofman,[9] the classification by discrete categories is preferable. A reasonable approach in such situations is to examine the risk over several discrete exposure categories and then, if the risk is approximately linear with dose, treat the relationship as a continuum. Mancuso et al.[5] and Kneale et al.[6] considered the mean dose in different groups as the exposure variables. Gilbert and Marks[4] noted the highly skewed nature of the data with only a small proportion of the workers receiving high doses. Fewer than 13% of the cumulative doses exceeded 10 rem in white males employed for more than 2 years. In such a distribution, the mean is a poor measure of central tendancy allowing a very small number of high-dose persons to dramatically affect the results.[12] In fact the positive results for multiple myeloma and pancreatic cancer are due to only 3 and 4 cases, respectively, with doses of >10 rem.

Another concern is with dose rate, which was not explicitly dealt with in any of the analyses. There is a reasonable possibility that the duration of time over which a given radiation dose is received may affect cancer risk, presumably with slower dose accumulation being less carcinogenic due to the opportunity for cells to repair. Given adequate variability in dose rate, this could be investigated in several ways, such as comparing cancer rates among workers with a given dose who incurred the dose in differing time intervals.

The effectiveness of radiation dose in carcinogenesis is another area of interest. Different effects of radiation doses received at different ages is a distinct possibility. This was addressed indirectly by Mancuso et al.[5] and Kneale et al.,[6] but their focus on cumulated dose failed to distinguish at what age the dose was actually received.[14] None of the cohort analyses considered this factor explicitly by differential weighting of exposure by age received, but several analyses did consider age at hire, which would be a weak proxy for the earliest age at which radiation dose began.

A more obvious factor is the differential effect of exposures at varying intervals before death. Clearly, a radiation dose received 1 week or 1 month before death attributable to lung cancer, for example, is quite unlikely to have had any impact on the induction of the fatal illness. The question of how far back in time the dose should be discounted is difficult to resolve since the true latency period (time between disease induction and death) is unknown.[13] Removing irrelevant exposures from consideration should remove some of the imprecision in the dose, refining the relationship of radiation to cancer risk.[15] Some attention was given to this issue by Mancuso et al. in all three of their analyses. Unfortunately, the question of effective dose was twisted into a question of at which predeath interval did cases of cancer differ maximally from noncancer cases. Stewart et al.[16] shed some light on this issue by showing that radiation doses began to diverge for radiosensitive cancer and noncancer deaths 20 years before death with a growing divergence up to the time of death. This is not, however, consistent with a 20-year latency as claimed, but rather would suggest a briefer interval between dose and cancer death. Both Gilbert and Marks[4] and Darby and Reissland[11] used a more flexible approach to the question and assessed the apparent radiation–cancer association under different assumptions about effective dose, as recommended by Rothman.[15] It should be noted that results for most cancer sites were affected very little by this procedure except for kidney cancer, where dose differentials occurred long before death and pancreatic cancer where differences were maximal closer to the time of death.[11] Gilbert[17] suggested consideration of a weighted exposure function defined by theories of radiation carcinogenesis.

Health Outcomes

This discussion focuses on cancer as the health outcome of interest, but there are several ways of classifying cancers. Essentially all the studies addressed the aggregate "total cancers," except for Kneale et al.[10] Also, most of the studies addressed specific cancer sites. One rather puzzling result of the analysis of specific sites is the failure of supposedly radiosensitive cancers, such as myeloid leukemia, to demonstrate any association with radiation.[18] The consistency across numerous other studies as to which cancer types are most readily induced by radiation makes the absence of an effect for cancers such as leukemia a reasonable basis for arguing against any cancer association with radiation in the Hanford data.

A useful categorization introduced by Kneale et al.[6] is that of level of radiosensitivity of the cancers. There is a tradeoff in any disease grouping scheme between maximum breakdowns into precise, homogeneous entities, and retention of statistical precision and power through an aggregation of a large number of the events of interest.

Organ system aggregates are often totally inappropriate since sites within a system may have very different etiologies. Similarly, lumping by location (e.g., Mancuso et al.'s "bone marrow" tumors for myeloid leukemia plus multiple myeloma) is not rational. The most relevant dimension by which to categorize (given that some form of lumping is needed) in a study of radiation effects is by radiosensitivity derived, of course, from external information. Although the means by which Kneale et al.[6,10] determined radiation associations is open to criticism, their rationale of comparing results from cancer sets defined by radiosensitivity is reasonable and would be of interest with the more conventional methods of Gilbert and Marks[4] and Darby and Reissland.[11]

Temporal Course

The temporal course of radiation effects and disease patterns must be considered to avoid spurious associations and uncover true associations. There is known to be an induction period between exposure to radiation and death, loosely termed latency. In order to effectively explore this concept, an analysis which explicitly deals with the time over which a person is observed is essential. The sequence of dose, latency, and effect over time has two implications: (1) Observation periods which differ in the relative amount of "latency time" and "effect time" will be different in the apparent risk estimates, that is, latency may act as a confounder; (2) The relative risk estimate should be observed from the "effect time" interval and not diluted with the "latency time." An example of complete disregard for latency is Sanders'[8] comparison of time trends in dose with time trends in concurrent proportion of deaths due to cancer.

Discounting recent dose is one mechanism for addressing latency. A more direct and informative way of asking the question about time course is to examine the relative risk for person-years of observation after different doses followed for different intervals. This allows simultaneous consideration of the dose received and latency periods, for example, in calculating cancer rates for those with 5-10 rem dose and 10 or more years latency. The time course of the relative risk across the dose levels as observation time passes can be directly evaluated. Only Mancuso et al.[5] attempted to address this issue in a comprehensive manner and other deficits in the analysis preclude definitive evaluation of the temporal course.

Two other factors fall under the rubric of time, namely calendar year and age. These are routinely adjusted for because disease rates so often undergo secular changes over time and manifest a strong association with age. The opportunity for error due to inadequate calendar year adjustment is il-

lustrated by the proportionate mortality analysis of Mancuso et al.[5] as applied
to lung cancer. Because the reference group was the 1960 U.S. population
and the lung cancer rate has risen so sharply over time, Mancuso et al.'s comparison of their cohort (with deaths concentrated after 1960) to the U.S. was
confounded by the secular changes in the lung cancer rates.[19] Aside from any
effect of radiation, the expected proportion of deaths due to lung cancer in
1960 was lower than in later years.

Surprisingly, only the two classic cohort analyses of Gilbert and Marks[4]
and Darby and Reissland[11] explicitly addressed age and calendar time in fine
intervals. Other workers such as Kneale et al.[10] considered proxy measures
such as year of hire. The case-control studies[5,6,9] failed to deal explicitly with
time at risk and consequently did not consider age-, calendar time-specific
period at risk. The Hutchison et al.[14] reanalysis of proportionate mortality
did include such an adjustment.

Statistical Methods

Two directly statistical considerations must be addressed as part of (though
not as the complete answer to) a resolution of the contradictory results of
these studies: power and multiple comparisons. Even with these issues, the
concepts are more important than the algebraic explanation.

Power refers to the ability to detect an association when it truly exists. It
is primarily a function of the magnitude of the association under the alternative hypothesis and the sample size. Several critics have noted that a study of
Hanford workers has very little power to detect an association between radiation and cancer under the currently proposed estimates of the dose–effect relationship. If, as Mancuso et al.[5] have argued, the carcinogenic effects of
radiation are an order of magnitude higher than currently believed, then
there would more likely be sufficient power to detect an association.[4]

Estimation of power is useful primarily to determine what magnitude of
an association one may have spuriously missed. Few of the researchers investigating the occupational risks to Hanford workers even touched upon this subject, when it would have been of great interest to know with what certainty
various magnitudes of risk could be detected. For example, with what power
could the BEIR[1] committee estimates be detected?

The other conceptual–statistical issue of some importance is that of multiple comparisons and its effect on the likelihood of incorrectly concluding
that an association was present. In a formal sense, the alpha-level is the acceptable risk of a type I error (incorrectly identifying an association), conven-
tionally set at 1 in 20 (0.05) or 1 in 100 (0.01). Consideration of many cancer
sites in many subgroups of workers obviously increases the likelihood of one or
more type I errors, that is, incorrectly identifying a chance association as a
true association. Prior specification of which sites are of primary interest
among which particular subset of workers obviously overcomes this concern.

This notion is really very intuitive—if there are statistical fluctuations in an array of numbers, some will appear (by chance alone) to be associated. Rather than formally adjusting for the number of comparisons, an adjustment ought to be made on conceptual grounds.[20]

If 50 cancer sites are examined and two or three are marginally "significant," depending on the sites which are positive and the level of the association, the overall conclusion may very well be that no association was demonstrated. The observed associations may legitimately serve as areas of primary interest in subsequent investigations, but it is not valid to determine which associations are of particular interest and test them in the same study (or in the same data set).[21] The argument often made against latching onto sporadic positive associations is that one is equally obliged to discuss negative associations, e.g., the apparent protective effect of radiation for certain forms of leukemia among Hanford workers. Hutchison et al.[14] noted that Mancuso et al.[5] found eight categories of malignant neoplasms with higher doses than the mean of noncancer deaths and nine categories of malignant neoplasms with lower doses, completely consistent with the absence of a radiation effect.

Anderson[19] graphically illustrated the spread of CMDs across the cancer sites, illustrating quite effectively that the dose deficits for selected sites are as striking as the dose excesses for other sites, a finding entirely consistent with sampling variability. Even Kneale et al.'s[6] data shows a great deal of variability in CMD by cause of death category, with cancers apparently less "radiosensitive" than digestive system diseases.

Hutchison et al.[14] pointed out several other errors by Mancuso et al.[5] related to the problem of multiple comparisons or more generally, using sampling variation to argue for positive findings. The doubling doses are based upon maximum contrasts in CMDs between victims of a particular cancer and persons dying of causes other than cancer. Clearly, the doubling doses contain a *systematic* error in that they were selected to be as consistent as possible with a carcinogenic effect of radiation.

Selection

Two forms of selection bias may operate in occupational cohort studies. The "healthy worker effect" describes the relative health advantage enjoyed by employed populations relative to general populations.[22] Presumably, healthy job applicants are literally selected to be hired and have lower mortality rates from certain causes than an unselected, general population reference group. Generally, coronary heart disease rates in such groups may be as much as 30-40 percent below the general population levels with selection against cancer-prone individuals less complete. Because of this, the proportion of deaths due to cancer is often higher among industrial workers than in the general population. The unique healthiness experienced by newly hired workers tends to diminish as time since hire progresses. It is generally acknowledged that this form of selection invalidates direct comparisons of working to general populations though such comparisons are useful in scaling the risk estimates.[11]

The obvious solution to this form of selection is to compare the health outcomes among differentially exposed subsets of the cohort. This refers to the comparison among Hanford workers, for example, on the basis of accumulated radiation dose. Instead of asking what the total cohort's cancer risk is relative to all U.S. white males, one asks what the risk is among persons with 15 + rem relative to those with < 2 rem, for example. This is obviously a major improvement in the accuracy of exposure classification over the implicit equating of "exposed" and "employed" inherent in general population comparisons.

Another form of internal comparison was chosen by Mancuso et al.,[5] namely, a comparison of radiation dose among those dying of cancer and those dying of other causes. This is essentially a proportionate mortality ratio (PMR) analysis as made explicit by Gofman:[9] the proportion of deaths due to cancer is compared across levels of radiation dose. The problem, as with all PMR analyses, is that relative (proportionate) excesses are not equivalent to actual risk excesses.[23,24] The proportion of cancer deaths, for example, may appear high only because heart disease mortality is exceptionally low. A clear illustration of this problem is the comment by Stewart et al.[16] that women are more susceptible to cancer than are men. While it is true that the probability of having had cancer among deceased females was higher than the corresponding probability for males, this is not the same as the (unconditional) probability of dying from cancer. In fact, approximately 4 percent of all males who ever worked at Hanford died of cancer while only approximately 2 percent of Hanford females died of cancer. Redmond and Breslin[25] concluded that an internal PMR analysis is likely to be inferior to an internal SMR analysis, the type of analysis reported by Gilbert and Marks[4] and Darby and Reissland.[11]

The second form of selection is selection within the cohort of later hirees[5] or healthy persons[10] into positions with higher radiation exposure levels. The Mancuso et al.[5] argument that early hirees have a low dose and high likelihood of dying due to a long observation period is invalid since a cohort analysis explicitly adjusts for the age and calendar time-specific period of observation.

If the postulated selection of healthy persons into high exposure jobs is complete, one can do nothing to adjust for it: higher radiation dose would imply healthier at hire, thus introducing a potential health hazard superimposed on a health protection (Burch, following Darby and Reissland).[11] Kneale et al.[10] chose to exploit information on internal radiation deposition as a surrogate for health selectivity within the cohort. Their rationale is that the healthiest job applicants were placed in the most hazardous positions, so that adjusting for hazardousness adjusts for selection. The only support for this is indirect, namely that failure to consider this index produces a strong negative association between radiation dose and total mortality. The measure of hazardousness that most effectively eliminated the association with total mortality was deemed the most effective method of controlling for selection though the apparent protective effect of radiation for non-radiosensitive cancers remained.

The possible existence of internal selection is indisputable; workers may very well be systematically assigned to positions with respect to their health. Nevertheless (1) the postulated selectivity has never been shown to have a strong influence on total cancer risk; (2) there was no direct validation that internal radiation monitoring corresponds to any known predictors of mortality and, in fact, Stewart et al.[16] showed that this variable was unrelated to cancer mortality; and (3) the coding of variables included in a complex multivariable model was arbitrary and not adequately explored descriptively. Variables appear to have been entered with the results guiding the decisions.[26]

A different form of internal selection relates to the selectivity in retaining employment.[12,27] It is hypothesized that (1) duration of employment is strongly correlated with radiation dose; (2) short-term employees are less selectively healthy than long-term employees, especially for noncancer mortality; and (3) therefore, due to these employment practices alone, higher dose (long-term) employees will manifest a greater proportion of cancer deaths. Their short-term (low-dose) counterparts are experiencing relatively more chronic cardiovascular and respiratory diseases. This line of reasoning is very plausible as a distortion in internal proportionate mortality studies. The recent analysis by Gilbert[27] indicated an excess of deaths from infectious diseases and symptoms and ill-defined conditions among short-term workers, but after 2 years of employment no cancer/noncancer differentials were observed based on employment status.

Alternative approaches to the same goal of adjusting for internal selection are worthy of consideration. One obvious method of examining the alleged selection is to tabulate cause-specific mortality by time since hire. Selection generally implies that the risk differential should fade over time. The pattern for coronary heart disease would be most likely to reveal selection. If groups within the cohort with different baseline risk were identified, an initial approach to the question of radiation and cancer ought to include a simple stratification to ask whether there is a cancer–radiation link within strata defined by their degree of selection.

Gilbert and Marks[4] noted a concentration of higher radiation exposures among craftsmen and operators, who were thought to be of a lower social class.[27] This variable was considered in the analysis and higher lung and prostate cancer risks among these workers were noted. These workers were not found to differ to any appreciable degree from other workers in their overall cancer risk. Craftsmen were at a 15 percent excess risk of cancer and operators at a 25 percent excess risk of noncancer deaths. Gilbert[17] mentioned the possibility that smoking habits or other hazardous exposures may differ in this group, but no supportive information is available. It should be noted that even a very small differential in smoking could greatly distort the estimated effects of radiation on cancer. Use of proxy variables for other cancer determinants (as Kneale et al.[10] did) is acceptable with adequate justification. Even then, presentation of adjusted and unadjusted results helps the reader to evaluate the results more effectively.

RESULTS

In summarizing the results of the various analyses, it must be kept in mind that these are not replications of a study but reanalyses of the same set of data. Inconsistencies are due primarily to the differences in methods.

Total cancers have been positively related to radiation dose in two of the Mancuso, Stewart, and Kneale studies and in Gofman's investigation. No suggestion of an association was found with the more conventional methods of Gilbert and Marks[4] or Darby and Reissland.[11] Given the most recent report of Kneale et al.,[10] it is reasonable to infer that all the researchers involved with Hanford workers would concede that cancer in the aggregate has *not* been shown to be associated with radiation dose in this population. The movement toward more similar methods and resulting congruity predicted by Peto in the discussion of Darby and Reissland's[11] paper may have materialized for total cancers.

Consideration of radiosensitive cancers as a group has produced positive findings by Kneale et al.[6,10] The more recent report used a more conventional approach except for the control variable introduced on the basis of internal radiation exposure. Nonetheless, results from the more conventional analyses (sequences 1 and 2 in their Table 4) reported by Mancuso et al.[28] indicate that only the introduction of control for "hazardousness" produces an association with risk of radiosensitive cancers. Given the problem of small numbers when focusing on specific cancer sites, this approach is promising, and while the positive results of Kneale et al.[10] are not definitive, they should not be dismissed. This is one outcome measure for which further analysis might be informative.

The only specific sites positively related to radiation exposure with any consistency and credibility are multiple myeloma, pancreatic cancer, and kidney cancer. Darby and Reissland[11] showed that the positive results for kidney cancer were due to one case with > 10 rem when only 0.01 cases were expected. This case obviously may have been radiation induced, but epidemiologic analysis cannot help very much in making that determination.

The situation for multiple myeloma and pancreatic cancer is very similar; any way one examines the data there are a few (2-3) excess cases in the high exposure (10+ rem) groups with no more than 1 case expected.[4,5,11,14] Statistics tell us only that these particular findings were rather unlikely to have occurred by chance had they been selected as cancers of particular interest before the study. Arguing for these cancers being radiation induced is the statistical significance and some external data[29] indicating multiple myeloma is inducible by radiation.

Arguments against a causal interpretation includes: (1) Many statistical tests were performed for many cancer sites and some would be expected (under the null hypothesis) to appear positively related to radiation. Other cancer sites appear to be somewhat reduced by radiation exposure (larynx, stomach), again consistent with an accurate null hypothesis. The reviews by the National Academy of Sciences[1] and the General Accounting Office[12] concluded that these findings are consistent with statistical fluctuations; (2) The major portion of the excess dose among pancreatic cancer cases was incurred within 10 years prior to death, inconsistent with most notions of expected latency for cancer induction; (3) These cancer sites have never before shown to be among the most radiosensitive; results for leukemia, which is most clearly radiosensitive, fail to corroborate the findings for these sites. In fact, Anderson noted in the discussion following Darby and Reissland[11] that the deficit in leukemia and excess of multiple myeloma may very well be a product of misclassification and (4) No dose–response gradient is apparent, only an excess in the 10+ rad category.[14]

CONCLUSIONS AND RECOMMENDATIONS

The many pages of published articles, letters, and replies directly concerned with studies of Hanford employees lead to the conclusion that excessive credence (from a scientific viewpoint) has been placed in this study. Anderson's conclusions[19] published before most of the reanalyses are very similar to those listed below; few substantive changes have been justified by the intervening work. One of the tenets of epidemiology is that replication is required for proof, since any one study has idiosyncracies and even errors that preclude firm conclusions. Replication requires a different population having different demographic characteristics, different diets, different smoking habits, and so forth, and not merely reanalysis of the same data. A single study should serve to move our thinking rather than convince us, with the magnitude of that movement dependent on the quality of the study. Many of those executing and evaluating this research appear to be swayed in direct proportion to their preconceptions. The evaluations seem to be working backward from the results to a justification or challenge of the methods rather than the reverse.

The invention of new methodologies [5,9] for these data is ill-advised from both a scientific and political viewpoint. In a study with weak or absent associations, a "new" method is not easily validated. A more conventional approach is to develop a method, test it with a known effect to demonstrate its validity and then apply it in a new setting. Liddell et al.[30] demonstrated quite convincingly the utility of case-control analyses of cohort data with the well-known carcinogenic effects of asbestos exposure. When a new analytic method is developed to address a scientifically and politically controversial area, it may appear that the method was "developed" with a particular result in mind. When more conventional analyses provide different results, as occurred here, the impression is supported. A careful, detailed movement from the conventional to a more novel approach is needed with discussion of precisely how and why the new method changes the results.

The conventional approach to cohort data has not been fully exploited. The temporal characteristics of latency period and the pattern of risk over time since exposure have not been completely explored. The outcome of aggregated radiosensitive cancers might be examined further. Nonetheless, the overall findings of no radiation effect on total cancers and a statistical association of radiation exposure with multiple myeloma and pancreatic cancer are rather convincing. Interpretation of both results must be in the context of other knowledge. Regulatory standards clearly ought not be changed on the basis of this single study. The particular effects in pancreatic cancer and multiple myeloma ought to be carefully addressed in future studies (not re-analyses). Our scientific (and regulatory) judgment should take note of these results. The epidemiologic study of cancer risks in Hanford workers is, after all, a very useful bit of information on the health effects of low-level radiation.

REFERENCES

1. NAS: *The Effects on Populations of Exposure to Low Levels of Ionizing Radiation: 1980*. Committee on the Biological Effects of Ionizing Radiation, National Research Council, National Academy of Sciences. Washington, D.C.: National Academy Press, 1980.

2. Radford EP: Human health effects of low doses of ionizing radiation: The BEIR III controversy. *Radiat Res* 1981; 84:369-384.

3. Land CE: Estimating cancer risks from low doses of ionizing radiation. *Science* 1980; 209:1197-1203.

4. Gilbert ES, Marks S: An analysis of the mortality of workers in a nuclear facility. *Radiat Res* 1979; 79:122-148.

5. Mancuso TF, Stewart A, Kneale G: Radiation exposures of Hanford workers dying from cancer and other causes. *Health Phys* 1977; 33:369-384.

6. Kneale GW, Mancuso TF, Stewart AM: Re-analysis of data relating to the Hanford study of the cancer risks of radiation workers. In *Late Biological Effects of Ionizing Radiation,* vol I. Vienna, International Atomic Energy Agency (IAEA-SM-224/510), 1978, pp 387-412.

7. Gilbert ES, Marks S: An updated analysis of mortality of workers in a nuclear facility. *Radiat Res* 1980; 83:704-705.

8. Sanders BS: Low-level radiation and cancer deaths. *Health Phys* 1978; 34:521-538.

9. Gofman JW: The question of radiation causation of cancer in Hanford workers. *Health Phys* 1979; 37:617-639.

10. Kneale GW, Mancuso TF, Stewart AM: Hanford radiation study III: A cohort study of the cancer risks from radiation to workers at Hanford (1944-77 deaths) by the method of regression models in life-tables. *Br J Indust Med* 1981; 38:156-166.

11. Darby SC, Reissland JA: Low-levels of ionizing radiation and cancer — Are we understating the risk? *J R Statist Soc* A 1981; 144:298-331.

12. GAO: *Problems in Assessing the Cancer Risks of Low-level Ionizing Radiation Exposure.* U.S. General Accounting Office, Comptroller General's Report to the Congress, EMD-81-1. Washington DC: US Government Printing Office, 1981.

13. Spiers FW: Background radiation and estimated risks from low-dose irradiation. *Health Phys* 1979; 37:784-789.

14. Hutchison GB, MacMahon B, Jablon S, et al: Review of report by Mancuso, Stewart and Kneale of radiation exposure of Hanford workers. *Health Phys* 1979; 37:207-220.

15. Rothman KJ: Induction and latent periods. *Am J Epidemiol* 1981; 114:253-259.

16. Stewart A, Kneale G, and Mancuso T: The Hanford data — A reply to recent criticisms. *Ambio* 1980; 9:66-73.

17. Gilbert ES: The assessment of risks from occupational exposure to ionizing radiation. In Breslow NE, Whittmore AS (eds): *Energy and Health.* Philadelphia, Society for Industrial and Applied Mathematics, 1979, pp 209-225.

18. Gilbert ES, Marks S: Comment on "Radiation exposures of Hanford workers dying from cancer and other causes." *Health Phys* 1979; 37:791-792.

19. Anderson TW: Radiation exposure of Hanford workers: A critique of the Mancuso, Stewart and Kneale report. *Health Phys* 1978; 35:743-750.

20. Schlesselman JJ: *Case-Control Studies. Design, Conduct, Analysis.* New York, Oxford, 1982.

21. Burch PRJ: Comments on "Radiation causation of cancer in Hanford workers." *Health Phys* 1980; 39:838-840.

22. McMichael AJ: Standardized mortality ratios and the "healthy worker effect": Scratching beneath the surface. *J Occup Med* 1976; 18:165-168.

23. Decoufle P, Thomas TL, Pickle LW: Comparison of the proportionate mortality ratio and the standardized mortality ratio risk measures. *Am J Epidemiol* 1980; 111:263-269.

24. Wong O, Decoufle P: Methodological issues involving the standardized mortality ratio and proportionate mortality ratio in occupational studies. *J Occup Med* 1982; 24:299-304.

25. Redmond CK, Breslin PP: Comparison of methods for assessing occupational hazards. *J Occup Med* 1975; 17:313–317.

26. Darby SC, Reissland JA: Hanford radiation study. *Br J Indust Med* 1981; 38:202–203.

27. Gilbert ES: Some confounding factors in the study of mortality and occupational exposures. *Am J Epidemiol* 1982; 116:117–188.

28. Mancuso TF, Stewart AM, Kneale GW: Analyses of Hanford data: Delayed effects of small doses of radiation delivered at slow-dose rates. In Peto R, Schneiderman M. (eds): *Quantification of Occupational Cancer*. Cold Spring Harbor, NY, Cold Spring Harbor Laboratory, 1981, pp 129–150.

29. Cuzick J: Radiation-induced myelomatosis. *N Engl J Med* 1981; 304: 204–210.

30. Liddell FDK, McDonald JC, Thomas DC: Methods of cohort analysis: Appraisal by application to asbestos mining. *J R Statist Soc* 1977; 140:469–491.

10.

Dose–Effect Models for Radiation Exposure

Marc Edwards

One of the basic problems in assessing or predicting the effects of low-level radiation is developing a model that accurately describes the effect of any particular radiation dose. Of the many types of models available for scientific applications,[1] the most useful are those that can be expressed in a precise mathematical form.

Although the ideal model would represent a precise simulation of the highly complex and multivariate reality of observed dose–effect data, considerable simplification is necessary to encompass and use the wide range of disparate results. As we shall see, the price of simplicity is loss of specificity and accuracy. It should be noted from the outset that dose–effect modeling is not a problem unique to radiation exposure. It is a problem common to a wide range of environmental chemicals and agents that are potential toxins or carcinogens. A recent bibliographic review article[2] listed more than 80 references on mathematical modeling of chemical agent dose–effect relationships. Indeed, we have the tremendous advantage of dealing with a single agent, radiation, and of having available a large quantity of data directly applicable to human exposure over long periods of observations.

FACTORS IN DOSE–EFFECT MODELING

The need for dose–effect modeling arises from several factors. For some types of irradiation conditions and organs at risk there are no available applicable data, or available data may be obtained from laboratory animals rather than from the clinical situation. Even when data are available, they may not span the dose range of interest. The most common example of this situation is the availability of high-dose data coupled with the unavailability of low-dose data, necessitating extrapolation to the low-dose region. Another common problem is the poor statistical quality of available data. As reviewed by Land,[3] in situations in which either the sample size is small or the expected effect is limited, the statistical uncertainty of the result can limit the usefulness of the data. One potential way around these problems is to develop a sound fundamental theory of radiogenic effects that would allow a theoretical, rather than empirical, calculation of dose–effect relationships. Unfortunately, the current level of understanding of these fundamental processes is insufficient for the task.

A basic assumption of dose–effect modeling is that the effect can be uniquely related to a single parameter, that of absorbed dose. This is a tenuous assumption in many cases, especially those encountered in irradiation of human populations. The process of getting from dose to effect is illustrated in Figure 1, which shows the induction of cancer to be the effect. Whereas the produc-

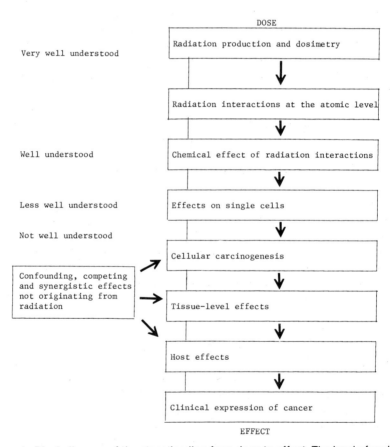

Figure 1. Block diagram of the steps leading from dose to effect. The level of understanding of the fundamental processes involved generally decreases as the complexity of system increases.

tion and interaction of radiation are well understood, the specification of only absorbed dose leaves much important information unstated. Other equally important parameters are type of radiation, its microdosimetric characteristics, whether delivered externally or internally, dose rate or fractionation schedule, size of the irradiated volume, and uniformity of irradiation.

Similarly, while the chemistry of radiolytic reactions is also well understood, the presence or absence of various radiation-sensitizing or -protecting agents can have a considerable affect on response. More research must also be undertaken to examine the radiolytic reactions in microenvironments that more precisely simulate those found within the cell.[4] At the single-cell level, a large number of empirical data, especially cell-survival data, are available. The precise nature of the biochemical damage and change induced in DNA is less well understood and is currently the subject of much investigation.

Again, many parameters in addition to absorbed dose are known to affect cell survival. For instance, cells are known to have various mechanisms of repairing radiation damage. If cell-malignant transformation, rather than cell killing, is the end point of interest, even less is known. Moving toward more complex biologic systems such as individual tissues and complete host organisms again increases the number of variables by such factors as immune response, age at time of irradiation, gender, and overall physical condition.

Finally, in many experimental and in all real-life situations, certain confounding, competing, or synergistic effects not originating in radiation exposure can severely influence the apparent results of irradiation. Two well-known examples are exposure to chemical carcinogens and cigarette smoking.

In principle, one can isolate the effect of absorbed dose from the many other possible variables by carefully controlling the experimental or epidemiologic investigation such that the only difference between irradiated and nonirradiated groups is the radiation itself. However, care must be exercised in applying the dose–effect model derived from one population to a different population. Clearly, the applicability of such a procedure will depend on the similarity of possible dose–effect-modifying parameters between the two populations.

STOCHASTIC VERSUS NONSTOCHASTIC EFFECTS

The radiation effects of greatest interest in dose–effect modeling are termed "stochastic." Stochastic effects are those effects for which the probability of occurrence, rather than the magnitude of the effects, is proportional to dose. Nonstochastic effects, such as cataract formation or gonadal cell damage leading to impairment of fertility, generally occur at much higher doses. Nonstochastic effects are proportional in severity to the magnitude of absorbed dose and may have a threshold dose below which no effect is observed.

In the case of stochastic effects such as genetic defects and carcinogenesis, not all irradiated subjects show an effect. In those subjects that do respond, the severity of the disease is not a function of dose. Owing to the probabilistic nature of the origin, stochastic effects are not expected to exhibit thresholds. The time sequence of expression of nongenetic, stochastic radiation effects in individual patients is illustrated in Figure 2. In this case, the histories of three patients, one a nonexposed "control" and two exposed to low-level radiation, are plotted on a time line. As indicated by B, all three are born at the same time. The nonexposed person lives for a given interval and dies at time D. The remaining persons are both exposed to an equal amount of low-level radiation at a single time indicated by X. Since radiation carcinogenesis is a stochastic effect, only two possibilities exist: either for cancer to develop or not to develop. Excluded is the possibility that all persons exposed to minimal radiation will develop "minimal" cancer. Hence, one exposed person continues with a normal life-span and dies at time D, which will probably be close, but not identical, to the nonexposed person. The other exposed person continues apparently unaffected until developing cancer at time C and dies prematurely at time D. The time interval from X to C, called the latent period, can depend on many of the variables previously discussed and is known to range from 5 to 20 + years.

Note that this analysis of the exposed, affected person assumes that radiation was the cause of the cancer. Since no effect can be associated uniquely with low-level radiation exposure, it is generally difficult to prove causation in individual circumstances. What can be observed is the excess cancers or

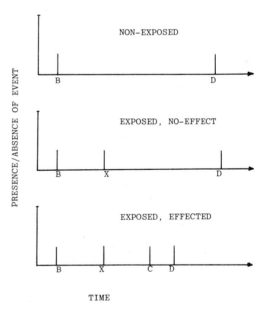

Figure 2. Schematic representation of the life histories of three patients. All were born at the same time (B), but died at different times (D). Two were exposed to identical radiation doses at time X: one patient was unaffected, whereas cancer developed in the other patient at time C.

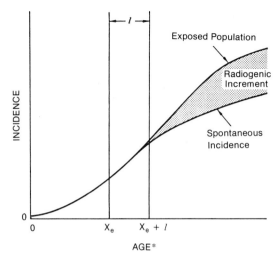

Figure 3. Cancer incidence in an exposed population, illustrating the excess cancer attributable to radiation. (From BEIR-III: *The Effects on Populations of Exposure to Low Levels of Ionizing Radiation: 1980.* Washington DC, Committee on the Biological Effects on Ionizing Radiation, National Academy Press, 1980. Reproduced with permission.)

cancer deaths in a population of exposed persons, as illustrated in Figure 3, in a comparison of the cancer incidence rates for an unexposed versus an exposed population. The difference in the areas beneath the two curves is the radiogenic increment, that is the number of cancers (or alternatively, cancer deaths) attributable to radiation exposure.

ABSOLUTE VERSUS RELATIVE RISK MODELS

As discussed by several investigators,[5,6] the relationship between the radiogenic increment and the spontaneous incidence can be expressed by two different mathematical models. The absolute risk model assumes the total risk (or incidence) of cancer R is related to the preexisting risk (spontaneous incidence), R_0, by the relation

$$R = R_0 + f \cdot D$$

where D is the absorbed dose (in rem) and f is the absolute risk per rem.

In the relative risk model the relationship is assumed to be

$$R = R_0 (1 + g \cdot D)$$

where g is the relative risk per rem. Unlike the absolute risk per rem, the relative risk per rem may vary with the spontaneous cancer incidence rate. In some cases, particularly leukemia, the excess risk is observed to return to zero after

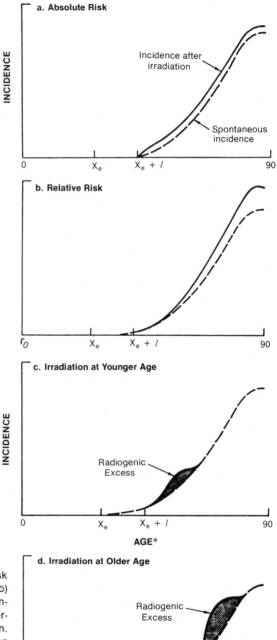

a. Absolute Risk

INCIDENCE

Incidence after irradiation

Spontaneous incidence

0   X_e $X_e + l$ 90

b. Relative Risk

r_0 X_e $X_e + l$ 90

c. Irradiation at Younger Age

INCIDENCE

Radiogenic Excess

0   X_e $X_e + l$ 90

AGE*

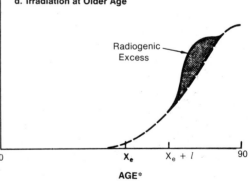

d. Irradiation at Older Age

Radiogenic Excess

0   X_e $X_e + l$ 90

AGE*

Figure 4. Possible types of risk models: (a) Absolute risk, (b) Relative risk, (c,d) time-dependent relative risk for two different ages at time of irradiation. (From BEIR-III: *The Effects on Populations of Exposure to Low Levels of Ionizing Radiation: 1980.* Washington DC, Committee on the Biological Effects on Ionizing Radiation, National Academy Press, 1980. Reproduced with permission.)

a period of time. This effect can be included in either the absolute or relative risk models by incorporating a cut-off time after which the risk is zero. If greater sophistication is desired, the risk per rem coefficients can be made time dependent, or more complex mathematical formulations of risk may be employed. A recent book by Gofman[7] apparently uses a gaussian-shaped time-dependent relative risk model. The various types of risk modeling, as illustrated in the BEIR-III report[5] are reproduced in Figure 4.

The mathematical model used to describe excess risk or radiogenic increment is, in principle, of little consequence because, for a given population followed for their complete lifetimes, all the models can be made to fit the data. Problems arise when trying to predict the outcome either from incomplete follow-up data or for one population on the basis of the results obtained from a different population. In the former case, one attempts to use present data to extrapolate or project to the future. Since the spontaneous incidence of cancer increases with age, the relative risk models predict a higher radiogenic increment than do the absolute risk models. In the later case, the assumption is generally made that the risk per rem (for either model) derived from one population is valid for some other population. Since the spontaneous cancer incidence rate is known to vary widely with location, socioeconomic status, dietary factors, and use of known carcinogens such as cigarettes, the relative risk model is again most affected. Until sufficient information becomes available to indicate a clear preferability of one approach, most studies will probably continue to use several outcomes.

Assuming that the total radiogenic excess is known for a range of exposures, it is possible to proceed to the dose–effect relationship. An example of experimental data for radiation induced mutations in a spiderwort plant *(Tradescantia)* is shown in Figure 5. This particular system permits almost four orders of

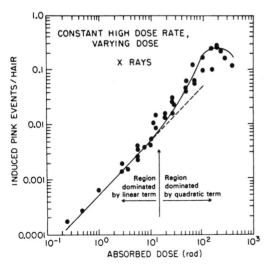

Figure 5. Example of dose-effect data from a simple biologic system, in this case radiation induced mutations in the spiderwort plant *(Tradescantia)*. Note that the absorbed dose covers four orders of magnitude. (From NCRP: *Influence of Dose and It's Distribution in Time on Dose-Response Relationships for Low-LET Radiations.* NCRP Report 64. Washington DC, NCRP, 1980. Reproduced with permission.)

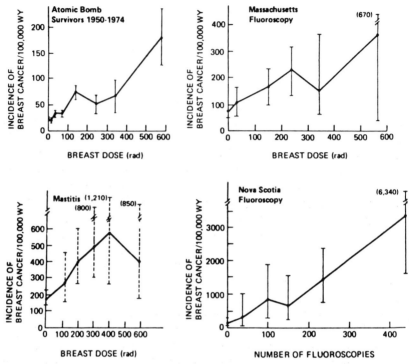

Figure 6. Examples of dose–effect data for breast cancer induction in humans obtained from four different populations. (From BEIR-III: *The Effects on Populations of Exposure to Low Levels of Ionizing Radiation: 1980.* Washington DC, Committee on the Biological Effects on Ionizing Radiation, National Academy Press, 1980. Reproduced with permission.)

magnitude in absorbed dose range with very little standard deviation in the response date.

Human epidemiologic dose–effect data cover a much more limited dose range and have much greater statistical uncertainty in the results. Representative examples are shown in Figures 6 and 7. The large diversity of dose–effect results for the same irradiated area, in this case the breast, is illustrated in Figure 6. In Figure 7, the dose–effect data for leukemia and breast cancer in A-bomb survivors are shown, using the recently revised dose estimates that have eliminated many of the discrepancies in results between Hiroshima and Nagasaki.[8,9] The general features of these and most other dose–effect data are lack of thresholds, an effect that increases with increasing dose up to a comparatively high dose, and decreasing effect thereafter, usually attributed to cell killing. The problem of the dose–effect modeler is to develop a mathematical function that both accurately fits available data and remains intellectually and scientifically reasonable in extrapolations to regions of unavailable data. As might be

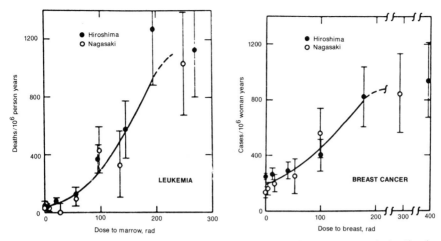

Figure 7. Examples of dose–effect data for leukemia and breast cancer induction in A-bomb survivors using newly revised dose estimates. (From Straume T, Dobson RL: Implications of new Hiroshima and Nagasaki dose estimates: Cancer risks and neutron RBE. *Health Phys* 1981; 41: 666–671. Reproduced with permission.)

expected, the latter task is more difficult than the former.

Viewed simply as an exercise in curve fitting, a general formula can be shown to fit most of the observed data.[5] If $F(D)$ is the incidence of effect attributable to absorbed dose D, then the general relationship is

$$F(D) = (\alpha_0 + \alpha_1 \cdot D + \alpha_2 \cdot D^2) \exp$$
$$(-\beta_1 \cdot D - \beta_2 \cdot D^2)$$

where α_0 is the spontaneous incidence, α_1 is the coefficient of the linear term, α_2 is the coefficient of the quadratic term, and the coefficients of the exponential term are used to describe the downturn in the high-dose region.

A discussion of the effects of low-level radiation need not include the exponential term, reducing the possibilities of the dose–effect curve to pure linear, pure quadratic, or a linear–quadratic combination. These various forms are illustrated in Figure 8.

One could also propose, although with spare epidemiologic evidence, a so-called supralinear dose–effect relationship in which the effect per rad increases with decreasing dose. When the various possible models are fitted to observed data, especially epidemiologic data, and plotted on linear–linear scale graph paper, as was done in Figures 6–8, there appears to be little difference between models. The wide range of dose, in this case from zero to several hundred rad, obscures the low-dose region, which is of greatest interest.

If, instead, the data and the dose–effect models are plotted on log–log scale

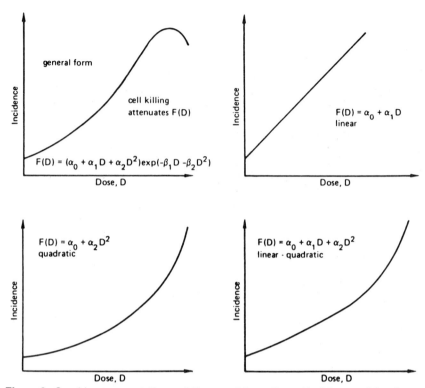

Figure 8. Graphic representations of the possible mathematical forms of the dose-effect dependence. (From BEIR-III: *The Effects on Populations of Exposure to Low Levels of Ionizing Radiation: 1980.* Washington DC, Committee on the Biological Effects on Ionizing Radiation, National Academy Press, 1980. Reproduced with permission.)

graph paper, as has been done in Figure 9, the low-dose region as well as the consequences of model choice become immediately apparent. Using artificial data points, but typical of those actually observed in low-LET dose–effect studies, Figure 9 is a schematic representation of the situation faced by dose–effect modelers. Here the pure-linear, pure quadratic, and linear–quadratic models all fit the known data in the 10–50-rad dose region. Note that on a log–log plot, the linear fit has a slope of 1, while the quadratic fit has a slope of 2. The supralinear plot is not based on any particular mathematical relation. Proponents of this "model" usually do not put forth a function purported to describe coherently the entire range of dose–effect data. Instead, they concentrate on the last few low-dose points and their local slope.

In any event, two conclusions can be reached: first, one cannot rely solely on goodness of fit as the arbiter of truth, because in many cases all models are equally adept at fitting known data. Second if one wishes to use dose–effect data in quantitative risk assessment for circumstances typical of average occupa-

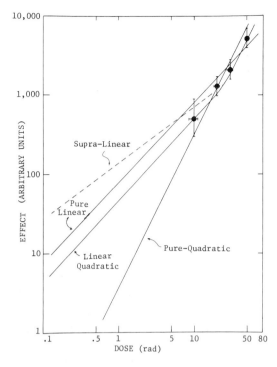

Figure 9. Schematic representation of the differences encountered in extrapolating the various dose–effect models to the low-dose region, using a log–log scale.

tional and medical exposures, the choice of dose–effect model could result in risk estimates differing by as much as two orders of magnitude.

APPLICATIONS OF THE DOSE-EFFECT MODELS

The empirical and scientific rationale behind the various dose-effect models has been examined by such groups as the BEIR-III committee,[5] the NCRP,[10] and the ICRP,[11] as well as by many investigators too numerous to mention. The supralinear low-dose extrapolation for low-LET radiation has been criticized for lack of substantial epidemiologic evidence, use of questionable statistical methods in its support, and lack of substantial radiobiological evidence for adopting it as general model applicable to a wide range of circumstances. Some animal experiments, particularly those investigating the effect of non-radiogenic parameters, have observed supralinear dose–effect curves. The argument is also made that especially radiation-sensitive subpopulations could give rise to supralinear effects. However, all national and international commissions and standards-setting institutions have currently rejected the supralinear model for use in risk evaluation of populations.

The linear–quadratic model, of which the pure linear and pure quadratic may be viewed as extremes, has a long and extensive history in describing dose–effect data. A very complete review of cellular, animal, and epidemiologic data and their relationship to the linear–quadratic model has recently been completed by the NCRP.[10] Much interest in this model was also stimulated by the microdosimetric theory of dual action proposed by Kellerer and Rossi.[12] As a descriptor of observed dose–effect data, particularly for simple biologic systems such as mutation induction in the spiderwort plant (Fig. 5), evidence for the linear–quadratic model is quite compelling. As pointed out by the NCRP and others, its applicability to more complex systems such as animals and humans is more problematic. Furthermore, there is increasing evidence[13] that a linear–quadratic dose–effect relationship might not be indicative of fundamental mechanisms responsible for radiogenic effects, as distinct from the position taken by the proponents of dual-action theory. Since the linear–quadratic model reduces to a predominantly linear relationship at low doses, the linear model can yield nearly identical results if only low-dose data are used for curve fitting (Fig. 9). It is therefore widely recommended that the lowest-dose data available be used in risk estimation in order to make the results less model dependent. The pure-quadratic model is most often viewed as a lower limit for extrapolated low-dose effects. Extensive evidence for its adoption as a generally applicable low-LET dose-effect model is lacking, although some arguments were presented by Rossi in his critique of the BEIR-III report.[5] Since those arguments crucially involved neutron and gamma components of dose received by the A-bomb survivors, presumably they will have to be reexamined in light of the extensive revision of the Hiroshima–Nagasaki dosimetry.[8]

An additional fact now becoming even more apparent is that there is no reason to believe a priori that a single risk-projection or dose–effect model can or ought to fit all circumstances. For instance, radiogenic leukemia appears to follow a curvilinear response, with excess risk eventually disappearing, whereas solid tumors often appear to follow a simple linear response with no diminution in excess risk over time. The shape of the dose–effect curve also depends on gender and age at time of irradiation. Thus, some models predict that more than half the radiogenic deaths would be attributed to that part of a population under 20 years of age at time of irradiation.

The shape of the dose response curve for low-LET radiations, particularly for simple biologic systems, has also been shown to depend on dose rate. This is illustrated in Figure 10.[10] The NCRP has estimated that the dose rate effectiveness factor (DREF), the factor by which linear interpolation from data obtained at high doses and dose rates overestimates the risk per rad of radiation delivered at very low doses or dose rates, is likely to be between 2 and 10. Although the qualitative and quantitative aspects of the dose-rate effect have been well documented in carefully controlled cellular and animal systems, the same cannot be said for human populations, primarily because of the paucity

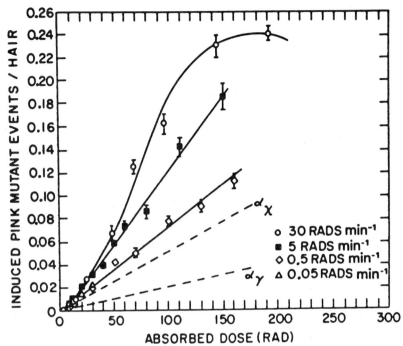

Figure 10. Effect of low dose rate on the dose–effect response of a simple biologic system. (From NCRP: *Influence of Dose and Its Distribution in Time on Dose-Response Relationships for Low-LET Radiations.* NCRP Report 64. Washington DC, NCRP, 1980. Reproduced with permission.)

of relevant data. The NCRP does conclude however, that "It would be most extraordinary if such dependence were not applicable to the same endpoints in the human being."[10] Even from this abbreviated discussion it is evident that the apparent simplicity of the few-parameter risk and dose–effect model is complicated by the realization that the parameters are not fixed, but instead must depend on a wide range of additional parameters.

Any modeling system requires careful examination of the intended application as well as the limits of applicability. One of the recurring problems with risk estimation and projection might be termed "multiplying a very small number by a very large number in order to get an impressive result." Thus, one could extrapolate the risk down to the 10-mrem range, multiply by the world population, and report that "low-level radiation causes 50,000 excess cancer deaths per year." Clearly, this represents a case of pushing a model beyond the limits of applicability. In recognition of this problem, the BEIR-III committee predicted effects only for a single exposure of 10 rad and lifetime continuous exposure of 1 rad/year, further stating that they neither knew nor would predict the effects of 100 mrem/year.[5]

An alternative chosen by previous commissions and committees is to embrace a "conservative" model with the qualification that the actual radiogenic excess will most likely be well below that estimated by the model. Unfortunately, the possibility that a model could be predicting only an upper limit is often ignored or forgotten.

A similar situation occurs in risk estimation for the purpose of setting radiation protection standards for occupationally exposed workers, as has been done by the ICRP.[11] In this case, since the intent is presumably to allow a margin of safety, and since the target population is comparatively small, the use of the simple linear model without provision for the possibility of modifying factors, such as dose rate, is quite defensible. Nevertheless, the use of such risk factors in evaluating possible effects to the public at large may be neither appropriate nor accurate.

A final situation, which might be encountered in a court case, is estimation of "relative attributable risk." As reviewed by Bond,[14] circumstances might arise in which a person with a known history of radiation exposure in whom cancer has developed would like to be informed of the probability that the cancer is radiogenic. This is a completely different situation from the one discussed earlier, namely, predicting the excess incidence of cancer in an exposed population. Relative attributable risk is the ratio of risk from one particular cause to the total risk from all causes. As shown in a sample calculation,[14] the relative attributable risk can be quite high. The linear dose–effect model would indicate that a person who received a 10-rad exposure and in whom leukemia subsequently develops might correlate with a 28 percent probability of radiation-induced cancer. Nevertheless, although such calculations are mathematically correct, they can be misleading in that the uncertainties inherent in the model from which they are derived are often left unstated. The example of attributable risk cited above is valid only to the extent that (1) the person is a typical member of the population from which the radiation and total risk estimates were derived, (2) the dose–effect model is valid and accurate, and (3) the person in question was not exposed to carcinogens other than radiation. When these factors are taken into account, the range of uncertainty in assigning relative attributable risk can be considerable.

CONCLUSIONS

In summary, several conclusions, both scientific and philosophical can be drawn. First, the process of radiogenic induction of a stochastic effect is complex at any dose level, and probably even more so at low doses and dose rates. Second, the magnitude, shape, and time dependence of dose–effect relationships are dependent on many factors other than absorbed dose. Some of these factors, such as appropriateness of absolute versus relative risk, may be determined by longer follow-up periods. Other factors, such as the effects of gender and age, may be resolved by more careful analysis of existing cohort data. However, the effects of some factors may never be resolved. Third, of the plausible dose–effect relationships, the current weight of evidence supports the linear-quadratic and linear formulations. Since these are identical in the low-dose region, it is commonly recommended that, whenever possible, only low-dose data be used in estimating risk. Finally, blind extrapolation of dose–effect models to very low dose regions is fraught with difficulties. The assumptions, qualifiers, and range of probable error of such extrapolations should be carefully stated. The "conservative" endorsement of a linear no-threshold model, in which a large enough exposed population will always yield an effect, carries with it the requirement that the scenario for exposure of such a large population be plausible and realistic. Increased understanding of the fundamental processses of radiogenic effects should lead to a significant reduction in current uncertainties. For the present, one must be guided not only by science and empiricism, but by prudence and perspective as well.

REFERENCES

1. Gorin G. The role of models in radiation science. *Int J Rad Oncol Biol Phys.* 1979; 5:1035–1040.

2. Krewski D, Brown C: Carcinogenic risk assesssment: A guide to the literature. *Biometrics* 1981; 37:353–366.

3. Land CE: Estimating cancer risks from low doses of ionizing radiation. *Science* 1980; 209:1197–1203.

4. Thomas JK: Chemical processes induced radiolytically in well-defined aqueous systems. *Int J Radiat Oncol Biol Phys* 1979; 5:1049–1054.

5. BEIR-III: *The Effects on Populations of Exposure to Low Levels of Ionizing Radiation: 1980.* Washington DC, Committee on the Biological Effects on Ionizing Radiations, National Academy Press, 1980.

6. Cohen BL: The BEIR Report relative risk and absolute risk models for estimating effects of low level radiation. *Health Phys* 1979; 37: 509–516.

7. Gofman J: *Radiation and Human Health.* San Francisco, Sierra Club Books, 1981.

8. Loewe WE, Mendelsohn E: Revised dose estimates at new Hiroshima and Nagasaki dose estimates: Cancer risks and neutron RBE. *Health Phys* 1981; 41:663–666.

9. Straume T, Dobson RL: Implications of new Hiroshima and Nagasaki dose estimates: Cancer risks and neutron RBE. *Health Phys* 1981: 41:666–671.

10. NCRP: *Influence of Dose and Its Distribution in Time on Dose-Response Relationships for Low-LET Radiations.* NCRP Report 64. Washington DC, National Council on Radiation Protection and Measurements, 1980.

11. ICRP: *Recommendations of the ICRP* International Commission on Radiation Units and Measurements: (ICRP) Publ 26. Elmsford, NY, Pergamon, 1971.

12. Kellerer AM, Rossi H: The theory of dual radiation action. In *Current Topics in*

Radiation Research, vol 8. Amsterdam, North-Holland Publishing Co, 1972, pp 85–158.

13. Yuhas JM: Intrinsic and extrinsic variables affecting sensitivity to radiation carcinogenesis. *Int J Radiat Oncol Biol Phys* 1979; 5:1117–1122.

14. Bond VP: The cancer risk attributable to radiation exposure: Some practical problems. *Health Phys* 1981; 40:108–111.

11.

Estimation of Cancer Risk Associated with Radiation Exposure

Jeffrey V. Sutherland

INTRODUCTION

The cancer risk of low-level radiation exposure has been a subject of substantial scientific, public, and legal controversy in recent years. While this controversy has often been clouded by emotional arguments, it has roots in well-defined scientific problems associated with estimation of the risk of cancer induction. This chapter is directed toward: (1) clarification of these problems, (2) demonstration of the capabilities and shortcomings of present methodologies for risk estimation for the specific example of breast cancer, and (3) indication of the direction of future research essential to improvement of risk estimation procedures.

The central difficulty in estimating the risk of low-level radiation exposure has been, and will continue to be, determining the shape of the dose-response curve in the low-dose region. Weinberg[1] has implied that this problem, while important, may be trans-scientific, i.e., may reside in the public and scientific community's attitude toward the issue. Figure 1 shows the history of radiation worker permissible exposure levels during this century.[2] These limits have decreased from 57 rads/year in 1925 (recommended by Mutacheller and Sievert) to 5 rem/year in 1957 (adopted by the NCRP). This decrease in permissible exposure levels was prompted by our ability to use radiation with less exposure and a real increase in the body of scientific knowledge concerning potential radiation hazards.

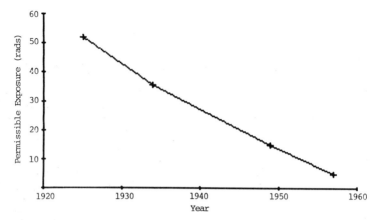

Figure 1. Recommended maximum permission occupational exposures for gamma radiation. Data from Morgan [2].

THE LOW-DOSE EXTRAPOLATION PROBLEM

The uncertainty of the shape of the radiation dose-response curve in the low-dose region is the result of ethical, economic, and experimental design constraints that force investigators to obtain data on in vivo carcinogenesis from (1) small-sample animal experiments using high-dose levels of exposure or (2) human epidemiologic studies which give relatively precise estimates of risk only at high exposure levels. Estimates of low-dose risk are generated by extrapolation outside of the dose interval where adequate data are available. Permissible exposure standards are, therefore, based on speculation as to the shape of the dose-response curve in the low-dose region.

An unavoidable consequence of this situation is that linearity versus non-linearity of radiation dose-response curves has been debated for decades.[3-9] Brown [10,11] has noted that radiation dose-response curves typically have a sigmoid shape but are approximately linear in the low-dose region. Linear extrapolation within that region is, therefore, appropriate. However, the same extrapolation procedure applied to data in the sharply rising midsection of the dose-response curve misleadingly suggests a threshold below which no response occurs.

Large-scale animal experiments have been proposed to solve the low-dose extrapolation problem. However, Schneiderman et al.[12] have noted that three million animals each in treatment and control groups would be required to assess risk at a level of 1 induced cancer per 1,000,000 population under the assumption of no spontaneous tumors occurring in the control group. Control of identification, randomization, and living conditions for millions of animals is extremely difficult. Spontaneous tumors occurring in control animals require increases in sample size of several orders of magnitude. Errors in handling and feeding, or loss of animals could produce enough random variation in the data to preclude identification of a small carcinogenic effect.

Even if a large population animal experiment were successfully completed, the problem of extrapolating risk from mouse to man remains. Animals used in such experiments are highly inbred and kept under carefully controlled conditions. Animal tumors are often morphologically different from human tumors at the same site. Growth patterns may be dissimilar from human tumors. Animal life spans are substantially shorter. Radford[13] concludes that "it is unwise to rely on dose-response data for cancer induction in experimental animals to support use of any particular dose-response model for human risk estimates from radiation exposure at low levels." Dethlefsen et al.[14] have strongly recommended that no further animal experiments aimed at quantifying risk per rad be funded and that research resources be directed towards experiments that elucidate the cellular and molecular events relating to carcinogenesis.

Turning to human data, Brown[15] has summarized the difficulties in using human epidemiologic data to assess risk at various dose levels. Humans are exposed to multiple carcinogenic agents. The dose levels and potential interaction between these agents are generally unknown. Measuring exposure to multiple agents over prolonged periods of time is usually impossible. The long latent period between initial exposure and the appearance of a tumor allows ample time for confounding factors naturally occurring in the human environment to distort findings. Genetic and environmental heterogeneity in human populations affects the shape of the dose-response curve.

Since available data are inadequate for direct estimation of risk of low-level radiation exposure, extrapolation from high-dose data is necessary. However, it has been shown[16,17] that even in the case of carefully controlled animal experiments, arbitrary selection of dose-response models can result in low-dose risk estimates differing by 5 to 8 orders of magnitude!

The difficulties noted above make it highly probable that no animal or human data will become available in the foreseeable future which will conclusively resolve the low-level radiation risk controversy. Experimental data derived from highly sensitive human cell culture techniques provides a promising avenue of research,[18] but such data will not provide accurate estimates of risk for free-living human populations.

THE RISK OF RADIATION-INDUCED BREAST CANCER

In order to examine the low-dose extrapolation problem in detail, it is necessary to focus on a specific cancer site. Breast cancer provides an excellent example because: (1) it is the most predominant cancer in females, (2)

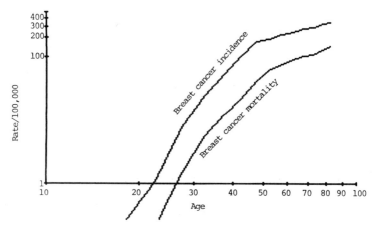

Figure 2. Log-log plot of U.S. white female breast cancer age-specific incidence and mortality. Data from Young et al. [19].

mammary tissue is highly radiosensitive, and (3) several recently published studies provide substantial new data on radiation-induced mammary tumors.

Breast Cancer Epidemiology

The best current estimate of the cumulative incidence of breast cancer in U.S. females aged 0–74 is 8.3%.[19] The cumulative rate is the sum of age-specific breast cancer rates[20] and is an indicator of the probability of disease over a lifespan. There is, therefore, an 8.3% chance that the average U.S. female will experience breast cancer before she is 75 years old. Breast cancer causes more deaths than any other cancer in U.S. females. Cumulative mortality for ages 0–74 is 2.6%. Because breast cancer incidence is much higher than breast cancer mortality (see Figure 2), the BEIR III Committee[13] recom-

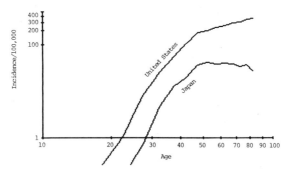

Figure 3. Log-log plot of U.S. white femal and Japanese (Osaka Prefecture) age-specific breast cancer incidence. Data from Young et al. [19] and Waterhouse et al. [21].

mended that incidence, rather than mortality, be used as an indicator of the impact of radiation on an exposed population.

Breast cancer incidence is dependent on geographic location. A highly relevant example for radiation studies is Japan[21] where cumulative breast cancer incidence during 1970-1971 in Osaka prefecture was 1.3% for women aged 0-74 (Figure 3). The low incidence of breast cancer in Japan is probably partially due to genetic differences in the population because descendants of Japanese who have migrated to the United States have only slightly higher breast cancer rates than women remaining in Japan.[22] The shape of the Japanese breast cancer incidence curve is different from the U.S. curve because of temporal trends in incidence, i.e., the younger Japanese are at higher risk than older persons. When curves from the United States, Japan, and other countries are adjusted for temporal trends the shape of the curves is virtually identical[23] (Figure 4), indicating that the disease is similar in all countries, but that risk varies with genetic background, diet, and other lifestyle factors.

Studies of breast cancer etiology must account for a wide variety of factors which have been shown to influence risk.[24] Confounding factors of age, place of residence, family history of breast cancer, and past history of

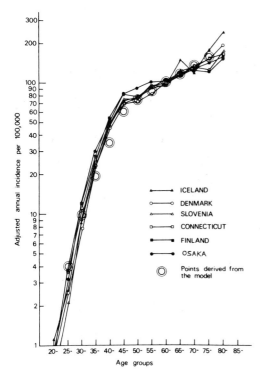

Figure 4. Shapes of breast cancer age-specific incidence curves from various countries after adjustment for temporal trends. Curves have been normalized so that the sum of the rates over all age groups is the same. Reproduced with permission from Moolgavkar et al. [23].

breast cancer have been shown to be associated with greater increases in breast cancer incidence than average levels of radiation exposure (150–250 rads) reported in most epidemiologic studies.[25] Socioeconomic status, age at menarche, menstrual history, and reproductive history can influence breast cancer risk to the same extent as these radiation levels.

Recent Concerns About Radiation-Induced Breast Cancer

Bailar[26,27] showed that the risk of radiation-induced breast cancer when using mammography for breast cancer screening of women under 50 years of age might be greater than the benefit associated with early detection of cancers. Using risk estimates developed by Upton et al.,[28] he calculated that 370 breast cancers could be induced for each round of screening of one million woman aged 35–39, assuming an average breast tissue dose of 2 rads per exam. An estimated 148 deaths would occur as a result of these incidence cases.

Mean dose to breast tissue at a number of breast cancer screening centers has decreased to 0.4–0.7 rads/view for xeromammographic techniques and can be reduced to 0.05–0.2 rads/view using screen-film techniques.[29] However, this reduction in risk from lower exposure has been partially offset by increases in estimates of the risk of breast cancer induced per rad of exposure due to accumulation of followup data on women in several major breast cancer studies.

Current Estimates of Risk of Radiation-Induced Breast Cancer

Recent followup data on radiation-induced breast cancer is available from three primary sources: (1) tuberculosis patients treated with multiple fluoroscopic exams, (2) Japanese atomic bomb survivors, and (3) patients with postpartum mastitis treated with radiation therapy. A recent study of Swedish women given radiotherapy for various nonneoplastic breast conditions is also of interest.

Breast Cancer in Patients Subjected to Repeated Fluoroscopies. In 1961, MacKenzie noticed radiation dermatitis in a Nova Scotia woman diagnosed with breast cancer. The woman's medical history indicated repeated flouroscopic examinations during the course of pneumothorax therapy for tuberculosis. After investigation of a group of women who received the same treatment in a sanitarium in Nova Scotia, MacKenzie[30] reported an incidence of 13 breast cancers in 271 irradiated women versus 1 case in 510 unirradiated women. Myrden and Hiltz[31] extended this study to include 783 female tuberculosis patients. Of those given pneumothorax treatment, 22 out of 300 developed breast cancer within 15–25 years of exposure compared to 4 cases out of 483 women who were not given pneumothorax treatment.

Reliable dose estimates were not available for these studies. The BEIR I Committee[13] reported an estimated average dose of 1215 rads and calculated a 0.78% increase in relative risk of breast cancer per rad and an absolute risk

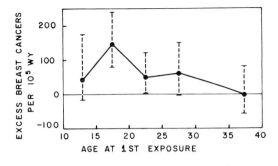

Figure 5. Excess breast cancer cases by age-group observed in fluoroscopy series with 80% confidence intervals. Reproduced with permission from Boice and Monson [32].

of 8.4 excess cases per million women years at risk per rad (henceforth, women-year-rad or WY-rad).

More recently, Boice and coworkers[32] reported on a series of 1047 irradiated patients in two Massachusetts tuberculosis sanitaria who developed 41 breast cancers in 10–44 years of followup versus 23.3 cancers expected. A control group composed of 717 women with tuberculosis who were not irradiated developed 15 cancers versus 14.1 expected. Expected numbers were calculated from age and calendar year using age-specific incidence rates from the Connecticut Tumor Registry. Assuming 1.5 rads per fluoroscopic exam, the average dose to irradiated women was 150 rads. The increase in relative risk per rad was 1.11% and the absolute risk was 6.2 excess cases per million WY-rad.

The fluoroscopy studies indicated that younger women may be particularly sensitive to radiation exposure (Figure 5), that excess risk did not appear until 15 years after the first fluoroscopy (therapy lasted an average of 3.3 years) and was still present at 40 years after exposure (Figure 6), and that

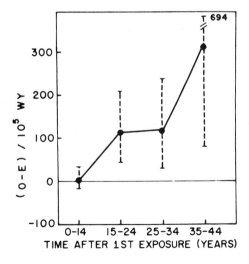

Figure 6. Excess breast cancer cases by time after time first exposure in flouroscopy series with 80% confidence intervals. Reproduced with permission from Boice and Monson [32].

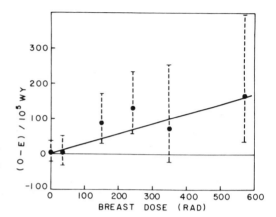

Figure 7. Excess breast cancer vs. dose in fluoroscopy series with 80% confidence intervals. Reproduced with permission from Boice and Monson [32].

a linear dose-response was reasonably consistent with the data (Figure 7). A linear dose-response implies that risk is directly proportional to cumulative dose. Schellabarger et al.[33] have provided data on mammary tumors in rats which lend additional support to this hypothesis.

The major uncertainty in the fluoroscopy studies, in addition to sampling variation, is lack of precise dose estimates. Although an elaborate methodology was developed to estimate dose, the time required for a physician to perform each exam is not known and this is the primary factor in determining risk to a patient.

Breast Cancer in Japanese Atomic Bomb Survivors. MacKenzie's work prompted Wanebo and coworkers[34] to study breast cancer incidence in Japanese women who survived the bomb. This work has been updated for the period 1950–1969 by McGregor et al.[35] and for the period 1950–1974 by Tokunuga et al.[36] The later publication reports on 360 cases of breast cancer occurring in 63,000 Japanese women. There were 288 of these cases residing in Hiroshima or Nagasaki at the time of bombing. Risk estimates for breast cancer in atomic bomb survivors have been lower than those reported in American studies, probably due to differences in genetic and lifestyle factors in Japanese versus American women. Loewe and Mendelsohn[37] have revised the dose estimates used in these studies based on corrections to Japanese building shielding factors. These revisions render previously published work out of date and eliminate some of the anomalies previously noted in the Japanese data.

Straume and Dobson[38] have examined the implications of the revised dose estimates. Breast cancer incidence in both Hiroshima and Nagasaki are now well represented by a single curve (Figure 8). Relative risk is reported to be 1.1 for a dose of 10 rads, 2.4 for a dose of 100 rads, and 4.4 for a dose of

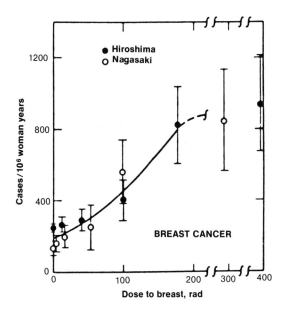

Figure 8. Breast cancer dose-response curve in Japanese atomic bomb survivors using revised dose estimates of Loewe and Mendelsohn [37]. Reproduced with permission from Straume and Dobson [38].

200 rads. Dose-response for a single high-dose exposure appears nonlinear. However, overall relative risk estimates for low doses are consistent with American studies. Absolute risk estimates are 1.4 cases per million WY-rad at a dose of 10 rads, 2.4 cases per million WY-rad at a dose of 100 rads, and 3.3 cases per million WY-rad, which are still much lower than those estimated from American studies.

It should be noted that since Japanese women have a low incidence of breast cancer compared to U.S. women, a similar increase in relative risk for both populations produces less absolute risk for the Japanese. In addition, absolute risk estimates depend on length of followup of the study population and are always low if followup is less than the entire life span. The maximum length of followup for the Japanese is 29 years, whereas some of the U.S. fluoroscopy patients mentioned above were followed for as long as 44 years. Finally, the Japanese sample consists only of women who survived until 1950 after abnormal exposure to radiation in 1945. This sample may be quite different from the U.S. population.

Despite problems associated with interpretation of the Japanese data, it is of interest that revised dose estimates produce a dose-response curve that appears to have a quadratic component. Since the Japanese sample consists of a substantially larger number of women with breast cancer in comparison with other studies, the Japanese data should provide the most precise estimate of the *shape* of the dose-response curve, even though absolute risk estimates may not be applicable to U.S. women.

Breast Cancer in Mastitis Patients Treated with Radiotherapy. In 1969, Mettler et al.[39] reported increased risk of breast cancer in 606 postpartum mastitis patients treated with radiotherapy in Rochester, NY. More recently, Shore et al.[40] followed up 571 of these women by mail survey. In addition, three nonirradiated control groups were examined to determine whether genetic predisposition to breast cancer, having mastitis, or geographic area of residence could account for high risk of disease in the irradiated women. The distribution of age, person years at risk, and length of followup intervals was very similar in the case and control groups. In addition, risk of breast cancer was similar across control groups so controls were combined in the analysis of results.

A generally linear increase in risk with dose was observed up to 400 rads (Figure 9) although the data are not inconsistent with a quadratic dose-response in the 0–200 rad region. The irradiated group was exposed to an average dose of 247 rads and had double the expected cumulative incidence of breast cancer after 32 years of study (Figure 10). Increases in breast cancer risk were found only in irradiated breasts and not in nonirradiated breasts in women treated with radiation therapy.

In this series, younger women did not appear to be at higher risk from exposure to radiation. The authors speculated that this might be due to the fact that breasts were actively lactating when irradiated. Serum levels of prolactin are highly elevated in postpartum women and prolactin has been shown to be a powerful tumor promoter in animals.[41]

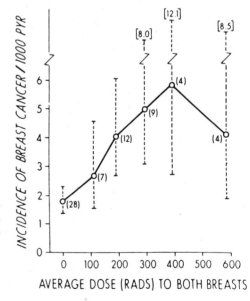

Figure 9. Breast cancer does-response curve in Rochester mastitis series with 80% confidence intervals. Numbers in parentheses are cases in each dose interval. Reproduced with permission from Shore et al. [40].

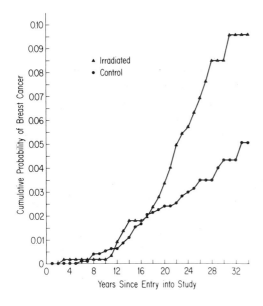

Figure 10. Cumulative breast cancer incidence in Rochester mastitis series by years since entry into study. Reproduced with permission from Shore et al. [40].

Increase in relative risk per rad was estimated to be 0.47% and absolute risk was 8.3 excess cases per million WY-rad. The followup period for women studied was 10–34 years. The minimum latent period was 10–15 years and increased risk was observed for the entire length of the followup period (34 years). Results were, therefore, very similar to results in fluoroscopy studies.

Swedish Study of Breast Cancer in Irradiated Patients. During 1927–57, 1115 Stockholm women were given radiotherapy for nonneoplastic breast conditions.[42] After followup for 6–42 years, 115 breast cancers were observed in irradiated breasts versus 28.7 expected. In nonirradiated breasts, 20 cancers were observed versus 19.9 expected. Median doses to the breast varied with length of treatment from 550–2000 rads. Doses in this study were much higher than those reported in American studies. The BEIR III Committee[13] calculated an absolute risk of 6.2 excess cases per million WY-rad from this series and concluded that since risk from this unfractionated-exposure study was similar to risk in fractionated-exposure studies, risk of breast cancer was proportional to cumulative radiation dose.

Summaries of Human Data on Breast Cancer Risk. Boice et al.,[43] Land et al., [44] and the BEIR III Committee[13] have provided summaries of the implications of studies discussed above. None of the summaries incorporate revised dose estimates for Japanese atomic bomb survivors. However, all have agreed that studies of American women are most relevant to assessment of risk from

**TABLE 1. NO. OF RADIATION-INDUCED BREAST CANCERS AMONG
1,000,000 WOMEN EXPOSED TO 0.01 GY (1 RAD)**

Age (yr) at Exposure	Linear Dose Response[a]		Linear Dose Response + Cell Killing at High Dose Levels[b]	
	Absolute Risk Model	Relative Risk Model	Absolute Risk Model	Relative Risk Model
35	234	312	307	425
40	202	288	266	391
45	172	257	226	350
50	143	226	187	307
55	115	191	151	259
60	88	154	116	208
65	64	117	84	158
70	42	79	55	108

[a]An absolute risk of 6.6 cancers/10^4 WY-Gy and a 0.42% increase in relative risk per centigray (rad) were used in the computation.
[b]An absolute risk of 8.7 cancers/10^4 WY-Gy and a 0.57% increase in relative risk per centigray (rad) were used in the computation.

mammographic screening, particularly since Japanese women have a much lower spontaneous incidence of breast cancer.

Major conclusions are: (1) risk is proportional to cumulative dose, (2) women under 20 years of age are at increased risk, (3) breast cancer risk did not decrease during the maximum followup times of any of the studies (30–45 years), and (4) the multiplicative or relative risk model is probably the most appropriate for assessing breast cancer risk.

The BEIR III Committee[13] concluded that the risk estimates of Boice et al.[43] were the best currently available (see Table 1). Since data on Rochester mastitis patients treated with radiotherapy suggested that a cell-killing effect existed at high doses, risk estimates were calculated based on both a simple linear dose response and a linear dose response plus cell-killing term. These risk estimates are higher than the estimate published by Bailar[27] in 1977. However, average mammography dose has decreased. The net effect is that risk from mammography is still approximately the same as the Bailar estimate.

Risk–benefit analysis of mammography screening is a complex subject which requires extensive mathematical modeling for meaningful results. Although many models have been proposed, the analysis of Eddy[45] represents the state-of-the-art in this field. A physical exam alone is estimated to increase the expected life span of the average 50 year old woman by 37.55 days. An annual mammography exam in addition to the physical exam increases

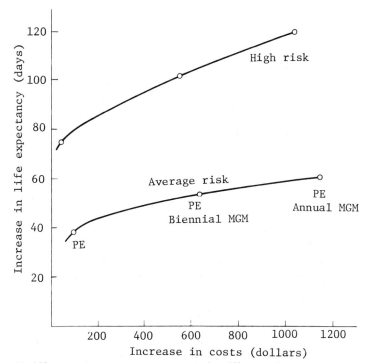

Figure 11. Life expectancy vs. program costs for difference breast cancer screening strategies in 50-year-old average risk and high-risk woman. PE is physical exam and MGM is a mammographic exam. Reproduced with permission from Eddy [45].

the average life span by an additional 23.05 days (Figure 11). Women at high-risk of breast cancer have about double the benefit in terms of expected increase in life-span. Radiation effects are estimated to decrease average life-span by 0.8 days in a 50 year old woman. Eddy's analysis is based on the assumption that each mammographic exam provides a dose of 1 rad to the breast and that 6 cancers per million WY-rad will be induced after a latent period of 10 years. The use of absolute estimates of radiation risk probably underestimates the radiation hazard. However, doubling the radiation risk decreases the expected life-span of a 50 year-old woman by only 1.6 days.

LOW-DOSE EXTRAPOLATION FROM BREAST CANCER INCIDENCE DATA

Radiation dose-response data from U.S. tuberculosis patients examined by fluoroscopy and mastitis patients treated with radiotherapy (Figures 7 and 9) are not inconsistent with a linear dose-response hypothesis, but both cases (see

TABLE 2. SAMPLE SIZE REQUIRED TO ASSURE THAT ACCEPTANCE OF THE NULL HYPOTHESIS OF NO INCREASE IN RISK IS NOT IN ERROR.[a]

Relative Risk	Cases	Critical No.	Sample Size
2.00	78	47	940
1.80	103	78	1241
1.60	158	119	1904
1.50	212	158	2554
1.40	306	226	3687
1.30	501	367	6036
1.20	1034	750	12458
1.15	1758	1267	21181
1.10	3776	2706	45494
1.08	5789	4138	69747
1.06	10097	7198	121651
1.04	22281	15842	268446
1.02	87397	61971	1052976

[a] Relative risk of radiation-induced breast cancer in an exposed versus unexposed group is listed in column 1. The total number of cases that must be observed to assure a power of 0.90 is shown is column 2. Column 3 indicates the number of cases that must be observed in the exposed group to reject the hypothesis of no increased risk at a significant level of 0.05. The cumulative incidence (0–74) of breast cancer in the U.S. is 8.3% [19]. The total number of women (half exposed, half unexposed) required to yield the number of cases in column 2 after lifetime followup is listed as the sample size in column 4. *(Adapted from Gail M: Power computations for designing comparative poisson trials. Biometrics 1974; 30: 231–237.)*

also the Japanese data in Figure 8) appear to have a quadratic component in the 0–200 rad region. While these data may be useful for establishing upper bounds on the risk of low-level radiation exposure, they remain inadequate for determining the precise shape of the dose-response curve in the low-dose region.

Consider the sample size requirements of an experiment designed to test the hypothesis that there is no increase in risk of breast cancer after exposure to low-dose radiation. In the fluoroscopy series, the estimated increase in relative risk per rad was 1.11%. In the mastitis series it was 0.43%. For ten rads of exposure, relative risk would increase 4.3–11.1%. To state with a 90% probability that 10 rads of exposure does not increase relative risk by 10% would require observation of 3776 cases of breast cancer in exposed and control groups, of which fewer than 2706 occur in the exposed group (using the experimental design of Gail[46]). Since the current U.S. cumulative incidence of breast cancer for women aged 0–74 is 8.3%, 45,494 women would need to be followed for their entire life span (see Table 2). If an increase of 2% in relative risk were under study, 1,052,976 women would need life-span followup. The largest currently available data set consists of 360 cases of breast cancer in exposed and nonexposed Japanese women. This sample size is only capable of detecting a 40% difference in relative risk between case and control groups.

IMPROVEMENT OF RISK ESTIMATION PROCEDURES

Precise estimation of the effects of low-doses of radiation (below 40–80 rads) requires extrapolation from effects at high doses. Such extrapolation requires a mathematical model based on relevant biological data. Future research should, therefore, be directed towards a more detailed understanding of the process of carcinogenesis and evaluation of mathematical models relevant to our understanding of that process.

The Multihit Model of Carcinogenesis

Dethlefsen et al.[14] have summarized the general aspects of mammary carcinogenesis in animals. Recent work[47,48] indicates that breast cancer induction in MuMTV-infected mice involves four stages. A cell undergoes mutation and then proliferates under proper conditions (promotional stage). A cell in the resulting clone then undergoes mutation and proliferates. Radiation may be involved in stages 1 and 3 (initiation), as well as stages 2 and 4 (promotion). Similar multistage sequences in tumor development have been observed in a wide variety of animal and human cancers.[49-51]

The multiple mutation theory or multihit model of carcinogenesis was originally proposed by Muller[52] in 1951. An extensive literature has developed from this idea during the past 30 years.[49,53,54] In the past decade, the multihit model has gained dramatically increased acceptance due to (1) Fialkow's demonstration that virtually all cancers arise from a single cell[55,56] and (2) Ames' demonstration that almost all carcinogens are mutagens.[57,58]

The present conception of this model[59,60] assumes that a normal cell is initiated (rendered potentially malignant) through alteration of cellular DNA by radiation, chemicals, viruses, or other factors. Initiation may be retarded by DNA repair or accelerated by promoting agents. Farber[61,62] suggested that a malignant cell is the result of an evolutionary process in which a normal cell and/or its progeny pass through several rate-limiting steps, some of which may be mutations. From a mathematical standpoint, "hits" may be either mutations or nonmutational rate-limiting events and the terms may be used interchangably. Breast cancer may be viewed as a four-hit process. The first and third hits may be mutations. The second and fourth hits could be epigenetic events that cause proliferation of clones of cells.

Recently, Holliday[63] unraveled two puzzling phenomenan that lend greater credence to the model. Many researchers have viewed carcinogenesis as an epigenetic process since programs imbedded in cellular DNA, which cause rapid prenatal cellular proliferation and which are normally dormant, could give rise to malignancy if triggered by mutation or other factors in the cellular environment. In addition, if hits cause malignancy, it was not clear why animals with short life spans are prone to tumor incidence similar to humans who have an extensive life span. Holliday proposed that "damage to DNA followed by repair can trigger epigenetic changes in gene expression which are responsbile for malignancy." Since DNA repair is more efficient in large long-lived animals, tumors occur over a more extended time span.

Tumor Growth After Induction of a Malignant Cell

After the induction of a malignant cell, tumors grow at a rate dependent on the promotional environment. It may require many years for a cell to produce a clinically observable tumor.[64] In the case of colon cancer, Sutherland and Bailar[65] have estimated that the time between a single initiated cell and an observable tumor is typically 21–40 years. This is the so-called latent period, a term used very loosely in the radiation research literature.

Minimum latent periods for human radiation-induced breast cancer were as low as 6–8 years at doses over 1000 rads (Figure 12). This suggests that at very high doses, cells may be rendered malignant and grow directly to form a clinically observable tumor 6–8 years later. Breast tumor doubling times have been observed to average 95.8 days.[66] Typical tumor size at clinical detection was 3.5 cm in a 1970–1975 study of breast cancers diagnosed in a

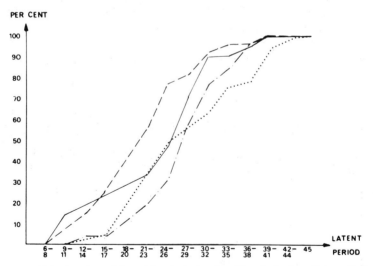

Figure 12. Distribution of latent periods by dose levels in Swedish radiotherapy series. Highest dose levels produced shortest latencies. Dose levels are 500-3999, 1000-1499, 500-999, and 1-499 rads, respectively. Reproduced with permission from Barel et al. [42].

Denver hospital. Approximately 35 doublings are required for a cell 10μm in diameter to grow into a 3.5 cm tumor.[64] Under the assumption of exponential growth, a typical breast tumor would require 9.2 years to become clinically apparent. However, tumors typically grow more quickly, often in half the time expected under the exponential assumption.[67] An average latent period of 4.6 years would be expected simply to provide enough time for tumor growth. The fact that median latent periods are greater than 10 years in all reported studies implies that in most cases, the radiation exposure begins, but does not complete, the process of induction of a single malignant cell.

Implications of the Multihit Model
The mathematical implications of this model are (1) cancer incidence increases as a power function of age minus the average tumor growth time, (2) age is simply an indicator of cumulative exposure, and (3) the slope of the curve of log incidence versus log (age − tumor growth time) is one less than the number of hits required to induce malignancy. Actual cancer incidence data departs from this curve due to artifacts induced by inaccurate reporting of disease (particularly in older age groups), changes in incidence of disease over time, age-related factors influencing disease occurrence, and exposures to carcinogenic agents at higher than background levels for portions of the life span.

Fitting the Multihit Model to Breast Cancer Data
It can be shown that the probability distribution of time to induction of a malignant cell is a Weibull distribution under multihit model assumptions.[65] Cancer incidence can be modeled by the Weibull hazard function since the hazard function is the probability of a cancer at time t, given no cancer before time t. Therefore,

$$h(t) = km^k t^{k-1},$$

where k is the number of hits required to create a malignant cell, m is the average probability of a hit, and t is the time from the beginning of exposure to the appearance of a malignant cell.

In order to allow for time between appearance of a malignant cell and clinical diagnosis of cancer (tumor growth time), we can make the simplifying assumption that t is age minus average tumor development time (4.6 years). However, in the case of breast cancer, females are probably at the same risk as males prior to puberty. This risk is virtually zero, since cumulative incidence of breast cancer over the male life span is 0.1%.[19] If we assume age at puberty averages 11.5 years,

$$t = \text{age} - 11.5 - 4.6.$$

Breast cancer incidence curves change slope dramatically at about the age of menopause (see Figure 4). However, we can fit the Weibull hazard function to the premenopausal incidence in Figure 4 and find that the number of hits required to induce malignancy (k) is 4 and the average annual probability of a hit (m) is 0.01091.

Fitting Postmenopausal Incidence Data

Two competing models have recently been fitted to breast cancer incidence data. Manton and Stallard[68] provide a model that fits U.S. female breast cancer mortality for 1969 under the assumption that both a pre- and post-menopausal type of breast cancer exist. Moolgavkar et al.[23] argue that breast cancer is a single two-stage disease with clonal proliferation between stages and that changes in the slope of the breast cancer incidence curve can be explained by variation in the number of breast cells at risk in the average breast at different ages.

The two-stage model of Moolgavkar and coworkers is consistent with observations in animal models,[14] whereas the Manton and Stallard model is not well supported by animal or epidemiologic data. However, the assumption that risk decreases at menopause solely because the breast decreases in size is not consistent with data which relate changes in endocrine function to cancer incidence. For example, radiation-induced mammary gland cancer in the rat can be substantially reduced by ovariectomy.[69] It seems unlikely that this affect can be accounted for simply by loss of mammary gland tissue. More likely, the combined effect of changes in endocrine function and reduction in breast size cause a decrease in risk. Let us assume that both of these factors reduce the probability of a hit at menopause, but that the disease remains a four-hit phenomenon consisting of two stages of mutation and two stages of clonal proliferation. The multihit model is analogous to the two-stage model of Moolgavkar in that a hit may be viewed as the probability of a mutation or as the probability of cellular proliferation after a mutation occurs.

An important implication of multihit model assumptions is that age is a surrogate variable for cumulative risk caused by continuous exposure to background levels of carcinogens. Peto et al.[70] performed an elegant animal experiment which provides support for this assumption (Figure 13). This phenomenon allows for a simple graphical interpretation of the effect on changes in risk on the shape of the breast cancer incidence curve.

It is obvious from Equation 5.1 that a large risk over a short period of time can generate the same age-specific incidence as a small risk over a large period of time. Fitting the postmenopausal data in Figure 4, while constraining the number of hits to be 4, produces an estimate of the probability of a hit of 0.00426. In order for this level of risk to produce the observed age-specific incidence of breast cancer at age 47.5, it is necessary to view this level of

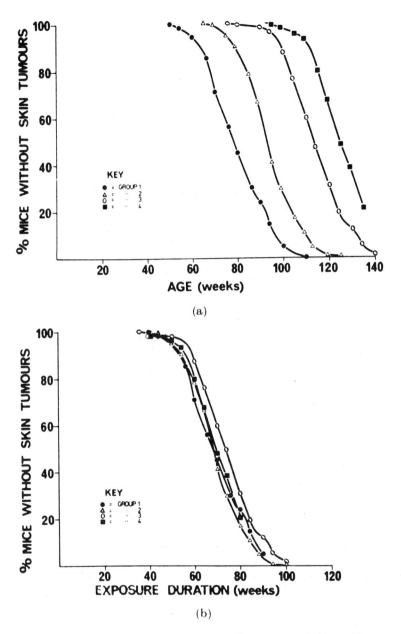

Figure 13. Life-table curves of tumorless mice after exposure to benzo (a) pyrene at various ages. Age and exposure duration do not affect the shape of the curves indicating that risk is a function only of cumulative dose. Reproduced with permission from Peto et al. [69].

exposure as occurring over (age − 11.5 − 4.6 + 78.5) years. Therefore, breast cancer incidence can be modeled using Equation 5.1 with,

$$m = 0.01091, t = \text{age} - 11.5 - 4.6, t < 47.5; \text{and}$$
$$m = 0.00426, t = \text{age} - 11.5 - 4.6 + 78.5, t > = 47.5.$$

This model yields a virtually perfect fit to the data. Changes in risk of a hit which produce an apparent change in the slope of the log incidence curve can be viewed simply as an expansion or contraction of time of exposure due to a decrease or increase in probability of a hit.

Introducing Radiation Risk into the Model

Consider now, adding radiation risk to the equation due to annual mammography exams. This has the effect of increasing the probability of a hit at the age that screening starts. It has an effect similar to menopause, but in the opposite direction. The slope of the incidence curve will increase, rather than decrease.

The effect of radiation exposure may be assumed to be proportional to background level of risk. This assumption is supported by the fact that increase in relative risk from a specific radiation dose is about the same for American and Japanese women, while the increase in absolute risk for the Japanese is lower in proportion to their lower level of background risk.

Figure 14 provides a graphic display of the effect. The shaded areas

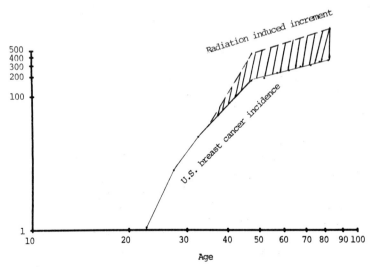

Figure 14. Log-log plot of U.S. female age-specific breast cancer incidence with hypothetical increment in risk induced by radiation exposure. Data from Young et al. [19].

represent additional breast cancers induced by the radiation hazards of screening. It is obvious that this model estimates higher risk if radiation exposure is begun prior to menopause, consistent with the findings of Boice et al.,[43] that risk is higher for exposure at younger ages.

A detailed analysis of the data on radiation-induced breast cancer in mastitis patients treated with radiation therapy and tuberculosis patients undergoing multiple fluoroscopies is beyond the scope of this paper. However, the model outlined above indicates the general method of approach. The cumulative incidence of breast cancer over the life span is the area under the incidence curve, or the integral of the hazard function,

$$c(t) = (mt)^4.$$

Since the probability of a hit (m) multiplied by time (t) is an indicator of dose, the model implies that the dose-response curve is curvilinear. If radiation only affects two of the four hits (perhaps only mutation, and not promotion phases) then the dose-response curve should be quadratic. If radiation affects cellular proliferation as well, the dose-response curve will be a cubic or quartic function. The Japanese atomic bomb survivor dose-response data (with revised dose estimates) are clearly nonlinear (see Figure 8).

SUMMARY AND CONCLUSIONS

Ethical, economic, and experimental design contraints force investigators to obtain in vivo carcinogenesis data from animal experiments or human epidemiologic studies which yield precise estimates of risk only at high exposure levels. Direct and precise estimation of low-dose radiation effects is not possible due to inherent statistical problems associated with extrapolation from high-dose data into the low-dose region. However, indirect estimation of low-dose radiation hazards is possible using the multihit model of carcinogenesis. This model is based on cancer incidence data collected over many decades on tens of millions of people. Available data on human radiation effects can be introduced into the modeling process without the requirement that these data precisely define the model to be used. This reduction in the information demanded from the limited data on human radiation effects allows a more rational approach to estimation of low-dose radiation hazards and helps to focus attention on research directed towards understanding the process of carcinogenesis, rather than on repeating human or animal experiments that cannot provide sufficient data to resolve the low-dose estimation problem. Assessment of the risk of radiation-induced breast cancer provides an excellent example of the utility of multihit modeling procedures.

REFERENCES

1. Weinberg AM: Symposium: Extrapolation to low doses of ionizing radiation. I. Introduction. *Rad Res* 1982; 90:33-34.
2. Morgan KZ: Cancer and low level ionizing radiation. *Bull Atomic Sci* 1978; Sept: 30-41.
3. Brues AM: Critique of the linear theory of carcinogenesis. *Science* 1958; 128:693-699.
4. Burch PRJ: Radiation carcinogenesis: A new hypothesis. *Nature* 1960; 185:135-142.
5. Shellabarger CJ: Radiation carcinogenesis. *Cancer* 1976; 37:1090-1096.
6. Yuhas JM: Dose-response curves and their modification by specific mechanisms. In: *Biology of Radiation Carcinogenesis.* (Yuhas JM, Tennant RW, Regan JD, eds) New York: Raven Press, 1976; pp 51-61.
7. Upton AC: Radiobiological effects of low doses: Implications for radiobiological protection. *Rad Res* 1977; 71:51-74.
8. Morgan KZ: The linear hypothesis of radiation damage appears to be non-conservative in many cases. *Proc IV Intl Cancer Cong Intl Rad Protect Assoc.* 1977; 1:11-14.
9. Gofman JW: Question of radiation causation of cancer in Hanford workers. *Health Phys* 1979; 37:617-639.
10. Brown JM: Linearity vs. non-linearity of dose response for radiation carcinogenesis. *Health Phys* 1976; 31:231-245.
11. Brown JM: The shape of the dose-response curve for radiation carcinogenesis: Extrapolation to low doses. *Rad Res* 1977; 71:34-50.
12. Schneiderman MA, Mantel N, Brown CC: From mouse to man — Or how to get from the laboratory to Park Avenue and 59th Street. *Ann NY Acad Sci* 1975; 246:237-248.
13. BEIR: The Effects on Populations of Exposure to Low Levels of Ionizing Radiation: 1980. Washington: National Academy Press, 1980.
14. Dethlefsen LA, Brown JM, Carrano AV, et al.: Can animal and in vitro studies give new, relevant answers to questions concerning mammographic screening for human breast cancer? *J Natl Cancer Inst* 1978; 61:1537-1545.
15. Brown CC: Statistical aspects of extrapolation of dichotomous dose-response data. *J Natl Cancer Inst* 1978; 60:101-108.
16. FDA: Food and Drug Administration Advisory Committee on Protocols for Safety Evaluation: Panel on carcinogenesis report on cancer testing in the safety evaluation of food additives and pesticides. *Toxicol Appl Pharmacol* 1971; 20:419-438.
17. Chand N, Hoel DG: A comparison of models for determining safe levels of environmental agents. In: *Reliability and Biometry.* Philadelphia: SIAM, 1974. pp 681-700.
18. Waldren C: Measurement of mutagenesis in mammalian cells. *Proc Natl Acad Sci USA* 1979; 76:1358-1362.
19. Young JL, Percy CL, Asire AJ (Eds): Surveillance, Epidemiology, and End Results: Incidence and Mortality Data, 1973-1977. *Natl Cancer Inst Monogr* 57, 1981.

20. Breslow NE, Day NE: *Statistical Methods in Cancer Research Vol 1—The Analysis of Case-Control Studies.* IARC Sci Pub No 32. Lyon: Intl Agency Res Cancer, WHO, 1980.

21. Waterhouse J, Muir CS, Correa P, et al.: *Cancer Incidence in Five Continents,* Vol III. IARC Sci Pub No 15. Lyon: Intl Agency Res Cancer, WHO, 1976.

22. Haenszel W, Kurihara M: Studies of Japanese migrants. I. Mortality from cancer and other diseases among Japanese in the United States. *J Natl Cancer Inst* 1968; 40:43-68.

23. Moolgavkar SH, Day NE, Stevens RG: Two-stage model for carcinogenesis: Epidemiology of breast cancer in females. *J Natl Cancer Inst* 1980; 65:559-569.

24. MacMahon B, Cole P, Brown J: Etiology of human breast cancer: A review. *J Natl Cancer Inst* 1973; 50:21-42.

25. Kalache A: Risk factors for breast cancer: A tabular summary of the epidemiological literature. *Br J Surg* 1981; 68:797-799.

26. Bailar JC III: Mammography: A contrary view. *Ann Intern Med* 1976; 84:77-84.

27. Bailar JC III Screening for early breast cancer: Pros and cons. *Cancer* 1977; 39:2783-2795.

28. Upton AC, Beebe GW, Brown JM, et al.: Report of the National Cancer Institute Ad Hoc working group on the risks associated with mammography in mass screening for the detection of breast cancer. *J Natl Cancer Inst* 1977; 59:481-493.

29. Shrivastava PN: Radiation dose in mammography: An energy-balance approach. *Radiology* 1981; 140:483-490.

30. MacKenzie I: Breast cancer following multiple fluoroscopies. *Br J Cancer* 1965; 19:1-8.

31. Myrden JA, Hiltz JE: Breast cancer following multiple fluoroscopies during artificial pneumothorax treatment of pulmonary tuberculosis. *Can Med Assoc J* 1969; 100:1032-1034.

32. Boice JD, Monson RR: Breast cancer in women after repeated fluoroscopic examinations of the chest. *J Natl Cancer Inst* 1977; 59:823-832.

33. Schellabarger CJ, Bond VP, Aponte GE, et al.: Results of fractionation and protraction of total-body radiation on rat mammary neoplasia. *Cancer Res* 1966; 26:509-513.

34. Wanebo CK, Johnson KG, Sato K, et al.: Breast cancer after exposure to the atomic bombings of Hiroshima and Nagasaki. *N Engl J Med* 1968; 279:667-671.

35. McGregor DH, Land CE, Choi K, et al.: Breast cancer incidence among atomic bomb survivors, Hiroshima and Nagasaki 1950-69. *J Natl Cancer Inst* 1977; 59:799-811.

36. Tokunaga M, Norman JE, Asano M, et al.: Malignant breast tumors among atomic bomb survivors, Hiroshima and Nagasaki, 1950-74. *J Natl Cancer Inst* 1979; 62:1347-1359.

37. Loewe WE, Mendelsohn E: Revised dose estimates at Hiroshima and Nagasaki. *Health Phys* 1981; 41:663-666.

38. Straume T, Dobson RL: Implication of new Hiroshima and Nagaski dose estimates: Cancer risks and neutron RBE. *Health Phys* 1981; 41:666-671.

39. Mettler FA Jr, Hempelmann LH, Dutton AM, et al.: Breast neoplasma in women treated with x-rays for acute postpartum mastitis. A pilot study. *J Natl Cancer Inst* 1969; 43:803-811.

40. Shore RE, Hempelmann LH, Kowaluk E, et al.: Breast neoplasms in women treated with x-rays for acute post partum mastitis. *J Natl Cancer Inst* 1977; 59:813-822.

41. Furth J: The role of prolactin in mammary carcinogenesis. In: *Human Prolactin.* (Pasteels JL, Robyn C, Ebling FJG, Eds) New York: American Elsevier, pp 233-248.

42. Baral E, Larsson LE, Mattsson B: Breast cancer following irradiation of the breast. Cancer 1977; 40:2905-2910.

43. Boice JD, Land CE, Shore RE, et al.: Risk of breast cancer following low-dose radiation exposure. Radiol 1979; 131:589-597.

44. Land CE, Boice JD, Shore RE, et al.: Breast cancer risk from low-dose exposures to ionizing radiation: Results of parallel analysis of three exposed populations of women. *J Natl Cancer Inst* 1980; 65:353-376.

45. Eddy DM: *Screening for Cancer: Theory, Analysis and Design.* Englewood Cliffs: Prentice-Hall, 1980.

46. Gail M: Power computations for designing comparative Poisson trials. *Biometrics* 1974; 30:231-237.

47. Miyamoto JM, DeOme KB, Osborn RC: Detection of inapparent preneoplastic cells by in vivo cultivation of dissociated mouse mammary gland. *Proc Am Assoc Cancer Res* 1975; 16:15.

48. DeOme KB, Miyamoto MJ, Osborn RC, et al.: Detection of inapparent transformed mammary gland cells in vivo: Recovery of nodule-transformed cells from virgin female BALB/cfC3H mice. *Cancer Res* 1978; 38:2103-2111.

49. Sutherland JV: The multihit model of carcinogenesis: applications to human colon cancer incidence data. Ph.D. Thesis, Department of Biometrics, Univ. Colorado School of Medicine.

50. Berenblum I: Cancer prevention as a realizable goal. Cancer 1981; 47:2346-2348.

51. Cleton FJ, Simons JWIM (Eds): *Genetic Origins of Tumor Cells.* Boston: Martinus Nijhoff, 1980.

52. Muller HJ: Radiation damage to the genetic material. *Sci Prog* 1951; 7:93-493.

53. Whittemore A, Keller JB: Quantitative theories of carcinogenesis. *SIAM Rev* 1978; 20:1-30.

54. Peto R: Epidemiology, multistage models, and shortterm mutagenicity tests. In: *Origins of Human Cancer.* (Hiatt HH, Watson JD, Winsten JA, Eds) Cold Spring Harbor, New York, 1977. pp 1403-1428.

55. Fialkow PJ: The origin and development of human tumors studied with cell markers. *N Engl J Med* 1974; 291:26-35.

56. Fialkow PJ: Clonal origin of human tumors. *Biochim Biophys Acta* 1976; 458:283-321.

57. Ames BN, Durston WE, Yamasaki E, et al.: Carcinogens are mutagens: A simple test system combining liver homogenates for activation and bacteria for detection. *Proc Natl Acad Sci USA* 1973; 70:2281-2285.

58. Ames BN: Identifying environmental chemicals causing mutations and cancer. *Science* 1979; 204:587-593.
59. Boutwell RK: The function and mechanism of promoters of carcinogenesis. *CRC Crit Rev Toxicol* 1974; 17:419-443.
60. Trosko JE, Chu EHY: The role of DNA repair and somatic mutation in carcinogenesis. *Adv Cancer Res* 1975; 21:391-425.
61. Farber E: Carcinogenesis—Cellular evolution as a unifying thread: Presidential address. *Cancer Res* 1973; 33:2537-2550.
62. Farber E: Sequential analysis of chemical carcinogenesis. Laboratory Workshop In: *Cancer Biology I—Etiology, Diagnosis and Treatment.* Aspen: Given Institute of Pathobiology, 1979.
63. Holliday R: A new theory of carcinogenesis. *Br J Cancer* 1979; 40:513.
64. Collins VP, Loeffler RK, Tivey H: Observations on growth rates of human tumors. *Am J Roentgenol* 1956; 76:988-1000.
65. Sutherland JV, Bailar JC III: The multihit model of carcinogenesis: Application to colon cancer data from the Third National Cancer Survey (abstract). *Proc Am Assoc Cancer Res* 1979; 20:77.
66. Steel GG: *Growth Kinetics of Tumours.* Oxford: Clarendon Press, 1977.
67. Mendelsohn ML: Tumor growth and the cell cycle. Lecture, Univ of Colorado School of Med, Feb. 18, 1977.
68. Manton KG, Stallard E: A two-disease model of female breast cancer: Mortality in 1969 among white females in the United States. *J Natl Cancer Inst* 64:9-16.
69. Cronkite EP, Shellabarger CJ, Bond VP, et al.: Studies on radiation-induced mammary gland neoplasia in the rat. I. The role of the ovary in the neoplastic response of the breast tissue to total- or partial-body X-irradiation. *Rad Res* 1960; 12:81-93.
70. Peto R, Roe FJC, Lee PN, et al.: Cancer and ageing in mice and men. *Br J Cancer* 1975; 32:411-426.

12.

X-Ray Examination for Breast Cancer: Benefit Versus Risk

Glenn V. Dalrymple
Max L. Baker

Cancer of the breast is the most common malignancy afflicting American women. According to the American Cancer Society, one of 11 women (9 percent) born in the United States today, will develop breast cancer in her lifetime.[1] Twenty-seven percent of all cancers in women and 19 percent of all cancer deaths in women are attributable to breast cancer. In 1982, 112,000 women were found to have cancer of the breast, and 37,000 women died from breast cancer.

X-ray examinations of the breast are of considerable value in the diagnosis of breast cancer. This may be especially true in the asymptomatic patient who does not have a palpable mass. These x-ray examinations, however, are associated with both a finite though small risk of induction of cancer of the breasts and an even smaller risk of death from cancer of the breast.

This chapter presents a brief review of cancer of the breast and discusses the value of diagnostic studies, including x-ray mammography; the benefits and risks associated with x-ray examinations; and the future potential of computed tomography (CT) and ultrasound as imaging modalities in the detection of breast cancer.

NATURAL HISTORY OF CANCER OF THE BREAST

Cancer may be defined as "a pathologic disturbance of growth characterized by an excessive and unceasing proliferation of cells."[2] A frequently used synonym for cancer is "tumor," which actually means swelling—whether associated with cancer, inflammatory disease, trauma, or other factors. Another term sometimes used for cancer is "neoplasm" (*neo:* new and *plasm:*

119

substance). Neoplasms may be benign or malignant. They are considered benign if they do not spread to distant sites and malignant if they do spread.

Neoplasms are not subject to the usual biologic controls governing normal tissues. Although a number of normal tissues (e.g, skin, gastrointestinal, epithelium, bone marrow, testes) have rates of cell division as fast as, or faster than, those of many cancers, normal cellular growth in these tissues is controlled by feedback mechanisms. By this means, the size of organs, the amount of skin, and so forth, are controlled. A neoplasm lacks these restraints for controlled growth. Originally, cancer was thought to be the consequence of a "single cell gone wild." There is now increasing evidence that cells undergo malignant transformations throughout the life of an organism. Immune mechanisms are important in that they survey the body for the presence of these transformed (i.e., cancerous) cells and direct cellular and humoral immunity mechanisms toward the destruction of these neoplastic cells. The spread of cancer, (i.e, the clinical appearance of cancer either locally or by metastasis) may reflect a breakdown of the immune mechanisms.

Before considering cancer of the breast the anatomy of breast tissues should be reviewed.[3] The breast is composed of a covering of skin and a centrally located nipple. Radiating inward from the nipple are ductal structures that connect to various lobules in the breast. Connective tissue, lymphatics, nerves, and other tissues are present between the lobules. Cancer may arise from the cells of one or more of the basic structures. Approximately 90 percent of cancers of the breast arise from the cells of the ducts and lobules. The remaining 10 percent derive from other structures.

While one out of 11 women in the United States will develop breast cancer during her normal life expectancy, breast cancer is not a chance event that occurs randomly throughout the population.[4] Rather, there is a group of patients who have an increased risk of developing breast cancer. A number of biologic factors appear to be associated with this increased risk.

Age is one important factor, as there is an increased risk of developing breast cancer with increasing age. For example, only 2 percent of all breast cancers develop before age 34, whereas 50 percent of breast cancers develop in the 55–74-year-old age group. More than 80 percent of all breast cancers occurs in the over-age-40 group. Cancer of the breast is typically a disease of sexually mature women. It is actually a different disease in premenarchal girls, and is quite rare.

Pregnancy is important in that women who have had their first pregnancy early in reproductive life or who have had multiple pregnancies have a decreased incidence of breast cancer, whereas women who have never been pregnant display an increased incidence of breast cancer.

Existing evidence suggests that the use of oral contraceptives does not seem to increase the risk of breast cancer. Additional data, however, are needed for complete evaluation of this most important issue. As the population of women using oral contraceptives becomes older, hence at greater risk of developing cancer of the breast, more definitive conclusions will be attainable regarding the relationship between oral contraceptives and breast cancer.

Cancer of the breast has familial aspects as well. Patients with mothers or sisters in whom breast cancer has developed are more susceptible to the disease. Also, patients who have had a cancer in one breast are at greater risk of developing it on the opposite side as well.

Finally, patients who have had excessive exposure to ionizing radiations, as well as to various other carcinogens, are at increased risk of developing breast cancer.

DIAGNOSIS

The most basic diagnostic procedure is self-examination of the breast by the patient. Probably 90 percent of all breast cancer is detected first by the patient. These palpable lesions will be ≥ 1 cm in diameter and will have been present in undetected form for 1-2 years. Physical examination by a physician may detect an additional few percent of breast cancers beyond those discovered by self-examination. Mammography can detect tumors well below 1 cm, and the prognosis for cure of these small tumors is excellent. In at least one major study, 45 percent of all breast cancers were detected by mammography alone. These tumors were not identified by physical examination before mammography.[5]

Thus x-ray mammography (film and xeroradiography) has become an important tool in the physician's diagnostic armamentarium for breast cancer detection. A physical examination is included as part of the mammographic study. Mammography by CT techniques may have even greater sensitivity and specificity than conventional film mammography, and this technique remains under investigation. Noninvasive modalities such as ultrasound and nuclear magnetic resonance (NMR) may have great potential for breast cancer detection as well and are under investigation. Thermography of the breast, unfortunately, has proven disappointing. Although safe and without x-ray exposure, thermography has not led to the detection of a substantial number of small preclinical lesions. Futhermore, thermography does not offer localization for biopsy and produces a high percentage of false-positive results.

In order to establish the definitive diagnosis of breast cancer, a biopsy of the suspected tissues must be performed. In some instances this is done by means of an incision, while in other cases a needle biopsy can be performed.

The preferred treatment of breast cancer is hotly debated. In general, at least 95 percent of localized ($\leqslant$ 1 cm) cancers of the breast are cured, usually by surgery. This percentage decreases to 40 percent or less for patients with nodal metastasis at the time of diagnosis.[4] Wide variations in the type of surgical procedure (the amount of tissue removed), the application of radiotherapy, and the use of various drug combinations are available; the optimum choice and sequence of these approaches can greatly alter the prognosis of disease in a given patient.

BENEFITS AND RISKS FROM X-RAY STUDIES

The greatest benefit to be gained from mammography is early detection of the tumor. As mentioned earlier, a cancer $\leqslant$ 1cm in an otherwise asymptomatic patient has a greater than 95 percent chance of cure.[4] This 1-cm size seems to represent the lower limit of detection by physical examination. As the dimensions of the lesion increase toward a more readily detectable size, the likelihood for ultimate cure of the disease decreases. A patient with a clinically palpable lesion but no nodal involvement has approximately a 70 percent chance of cure; with nodal involvement, the chance of cure drops to 40 percent. These figures are based on 10-year survival of the population studied.[4]

While the above factors seem to suggest that considerable benefit is derived from x-ray mammography, some problems must be considered. Mammography rarely provides an absolute diagnosis. False-positive examinations occur in which a study is considered positive but is ultimately proved negative. In the American Cancer Society–National Center Institute (ACS–NCI) funded Breast Cancer Detection Demonstration Projects (BC-DDP) study, 271,984 women were screened for breast cancer. Biopsies were recommended in 10,356 (3.8 percent) and actually performed in 5569 (2 percent) of the cases. In these 10,356 positive mammography cases, pathology ultimately confirmed 952 cases of cancer, or approximately 10 percent of the total positive findings.[6]

Another area of the BCDDP study has been discussed by Lester.[7] Approximately one-half the patients in the program are women between the ages of 35 and 49. Of the total cancers with diagnostic modality reports (901), 246 were found in women under the age of 50. In other words, 27 percent of the cancers found occurred in the 50 percent of women in the under-50 age group, representing a sizable yield of breast cancers in a group of women who would otherwise have long life expectancy.

The diagnostic modality breakdown in this group of women is also impressive. Of the proven cancers, 106 were found by mammography alone. An additional 118 were found by both physical examination and mammography. In 22 cases, the physical examination was positive while mammography was negative. This finding represents a 9 percent false-negative rate for mammography, as opposed to a 90 percent true-positive rate. On the other hand, the true-positive rate for physical examination was approximately 56 percent in women with proven breast cancer, while the false-negative rate was approximately 43 percent. The 106 cases diagnosed by mammography alone would not have led to surgery had mammography not been performed.

The major problem associated with mammography is the induction of new cancer. As with any exposure to ionizing radiation, there is an associated increased risk of cancer, and thus cancer death. Several populations have been studied extensively for breast cancer induction associated with radiation exposure. These groups include the Japanese victims of the atomic bombings and different groups of women exposed for a variety of nonneoplastic diseases of the breast. Boice et al.[8] have drawn several conclusions regarding these groups: (1) the risk is greatest for persons exposed as adolescents, although exposure at any age carries some risk; (2) the dose–response relationship is consistent wtih linearity in all studies; (3) direct evidence of cancer risk at doses of < 50 rad is apparent among A-bomb survivors; (4) neither fractionation nor time since exposure within the time limits of the study appear to diminish risk; (5) the interval between exposure and the clinical appearance of radiogenic breast cancer may be mediated by hormonal or other age-related factors, but is unrelated to dose; and (6) age-specific absolute risk estimates for all studies are remarkably similar. Finally, Boice and associates conclude that the best estimate of risk among Americans exposed after age 20 is 6.6 excess cancers per 10^6 women per year per rad. Parenthetically, it should be noted that these conclusions and figures are the basis for most of the breast cancer findings of the NAS Committee on the Biological Effects of Ionizing Radiation (BEIR-III).[9]

The value of 6.6 cases per 10^6 women per year per rad may be used to arrive at some estimates of risk versus benefit associated with x-ray mammography.[10] Assume a population of 100,000 women with an average age of 50 years. In current screen-film techniques, the average exposure per breast is 500 mR. For our calculation, we will assume 1 R total exposure for the procedure. The number of breast cancers induced in 100,000 women if each patient receives a mammographic examination may be estimated as follows:

$$\text{Number of breast cancers} = \frac{6.6 \text{ cancers} \,(1.0 \text{ R}) \,(10^5 \text{ persons}) \,(30 \text{ years})}{10^6 \text{ persons} \cdot \text{year} \cdot \text{R}}$$
$$= 19.8 \text{ cancers}$$

where the expected life-span of the irradiated population is an estimated 30 years and radiation is expected to induce 6.6 breast cancers per year after exposure of 1 million women to 1 R radiation. Of course, some of the radiation-induced cancers will be detected and cured at an early stage. With a conservative 50 percent cure rate, only 10 cancer deaths can be attributed to the radiation exposure of the population. This, then, is the risk of mammography.

Similarly, a benefit estimate may be computed for mammography. For the same 100,000 women and an overall incidence of 9 percent for spontaneous breast cancer, 9,000 cases of breast cancer would be expected to develop in this population. With a detection rate of 45 percent for mammography alone, and with the assumption that the tumors so detected are small and thus highly curable (95%), approximately 3850 cancers will be detected, treated, and cured as a result of mammography. Tumors not detected by mammography might yield a conservative 50 percent cure rate, providing an additional 2500 cures. Hence a total of 6400 "cures" out of 9000 breast cancers occurs in the population receiving mammography. In an equivalent population not receiving mammography the same 50 percent cure rate yields approximately 4500 women "cured" of their disease. Hence, the use of mammography adds approximately 1900 cures from breast cancer while inducing some 10 additional cases of breast cancer as a result of its use.

The above calculation has obviously used generalities. Nevertheless, from the risk/benefit position, the value of mammography appears significant. One factor, namely population age, should be mentioned as capable of altering this computation significantly. Also, the persistent reduction in radiation dose to increasingly lower levels in mammography decreases the risk of radiation-induced breast cancer from mammography.

The age of the population undergoing mammographic examinations significantly alters the risk/benefit situation. Computations similar to those described above performed for various age groups can be used to determine age-specific risk/benefit ratios for mammography. These recommendations have been published by the American Cancer Society.[4] The ACS guidelines recommend annual screening for all women over 50 years of age. For women in the 35-49 age group, two baseline studies are recommended between the ages of 35 and 40 years, followed by further studies as needed. Between the ages of 25 and 34, mammograms are recommended only when there is a family history of breast cancer or a reason to suspect the presence of pathology. X-ray examinations of the breast are not recommended for patients under 25 years of age. These recommended guidelines apply to the general population only. For those women at higher risk of breast cancer because of family history or other reasons, the physician must handle each case on an individual basis regarding risk and benefit.

For the future, the risk/benefit balance in mammography appears promising. Increasingly sensitive film/screen combinations permit a significant reduction in patient dose. X-ray mammography employing CT techniques holds some promise, although initial efforts have been disappointing. Ultrasound methods for breast examination eventually may develop detection rates approaching those achieved with x-ray films. Newer systems are being developed in an effort to enhance the value of ultrasound. Currently, some physicians believe ultrasound to be quite effective, while others do not consider the technique sufficiently sensitive. Nuclear magnetic resonance imaging is in its infancy, but ultimately may also be helpful in detecting breast cancer. Both NMR and ultrasound do not require ionizing radiation. Currently, conventional x-ray mammography using dose-reduction techniques appears to be the best diagnostic aid in the detection and diagnosis of breast cancer.

REFERENCES

1. *Cancer Facts and Figures, 1982*: New York, American Cancer Society, 1981.
2. Meissner WA, Diamonopoulos GT. Neoplasia. In Anderson WAD, Kissane JM, (eds): *Pathology*. St. Louis, CV Mosby, 1977.
3. Townsend CM, Jr: Breast lumps. *Clin Symp* 1980; 32:1-32.
4. Leis HP Jr: *The Diagnosis of Breast Cancer*. New York, American Cancer Society, 1977.
5. Strax P. *Early Detection: Breast Cancer is Curable*. New York, New American Library, 1974.
6. Upton AC: Risks of mammography. Report to the National Cancer Institute. July 8, 1976.
7. Lester RG. Risk versus benefit in mammography. *Radiology* 1977; 124: 1-6.
8. Boice JD, Land CE, Shore RE, et al: Risk of breast cancer following low-dose radiation exposure. *Radiology* 1979; 131: 589-597.
9. BEIR: Committe on the Biological Effects of Ionizing Radiation, *The Effects on Populations of Exposures to Low Levels of Ionizing Radiation: 1980.* Washington DC, National Academy Press, 1980.
10. Letton AH, Wilson JP, Mason EM: The value of breast cancer screening in women less than fifty years of age. *Cancer* 1977; 40: 1-3.

13.

Radiation and the Fetus

Max L. Baker
Glenn V. Dalrymple

One of the basic rules or "laws" of radiation biology is the law of Bergonie and Tribondeau. This law states that cells undergoing rapid division and that are poorly differentiated (i.e., poorly specialized) are most sensitive to radiation.[1] These properties describe very well the cells of the developing embryo and fetus. The embryo and fetus are characterized by cell populations that are rapidly dividing and, for the most part, poorly differentiated. Thus the fetus and embryo represent a very special and radiation-sensitive entity. To clarify terms, in human embryology the embryo exists from the moment of fertilization to the end of the eighth week after fertilization. The term fetus is then used to describe the unborn organism from the ninth week until birth.[2]

Before we pursue the radiation sensitivity of the young organism, some discussion of the time sequence of gestation is important, because the timing of radiation exposure during pregnancy is critical to considering possible effects of the radiation. Ovulation takes place in the middle of the menstrual cycle, about day 14. The day of conception is day 0 of gestation. The fertilized egg, or zygote, undergoes multiple divisions as an embryo and implants in the uterine wall at about day 10–12 of the gestational period. After implantation, the process of organ development (organogenesis) begins. This process takes place on a very tightly scheduled basis through the next several weeks and is essentially complete by about day 50 of gestation. From this point, the fetus simply grows larger throughout the remainder of gestation.[2]

Radiation exposure before implantation generally results in an all-or-nothing response, meaning that the pregnancy either terminates with resorption of the embryo or proceeds with no apparent problems.[3] The percentage of prenatal death (before implantation) declines very rapidly after the first week or so of pregnancy.[4] The likelihood of in utero death after implantation is small. Even during the preimplantation time, doses on the order of 100 rad are usually required to cause embryonic death.

As mentioned earlier, organ systems begin to develop immediately after implantation of the embryo in the uterine wall. This period of organogenesis represents the most sensitive time of fetal life.[5] Beginning with implantation, the fetus becomes increasingly sensitive to the induction of congenital anomalies (i.e., birth defects) until peak sensitivity is reached somewhere around day 28–30 of gestation. Very low radiation doses during this time period have a finite likelihood of producing visible congenital abnormalities. The specific anomaly produced depends on the specific point during organogenesis that the radiation exposure was delivered.[5] After the period of peak sensitivity during organogenesis, the radiation sensitivity of the fetus declines from the standpoint of congenitally induced anomalies. Radiation-induced developmental anomalies remain a distinct possibility, however, throughout the gestational period. The developing central nervous system (CNS) remains sensitive to radiation throughout gestation, and perhaps into the first few months of life. For example, a number of children in utero at the time of the atomic bombings in Japan have exhibited such anomalies, including microcephaly and deficiencies of the CNS as a result of the radiation exposure.[6] The radiation doses to these children were in the range of ≥50 rad.

Generally, radiation exposures in the latter part of gestation do not produce gross congenital anomalies or fetal death. Exposures during this latter part of gestation, as well as during the very early period of gestation (before implantation) can produce an overall stunting of growth in the irradiated person. Although the physical size of the person may be somewhat reduced, he or she remains physically normal in other ways. It may be prudent to mention that all the anomalies reportedly caused by human fetal irradiation have been confirmed experimentally in the mouse or rat when they could be recognized and analyzed.[4]

Another area of concern in regard to radiation and the fetus is the induction of cancer. While there is controversy over this issue, it may be that the fetus is extremely susceptible to the induction of cancer. Data suggest that in utero radiation exposure may increase the likelihood of early childhood cancer by as much as 50 percent, and perhaps more.[7] The cancers primarily involved are leukemia and tumors of the CNS. Radiation exposure during the first trimester appears more likely to result in cancer induction than in the second or third trimester.

To summarize radiation effects on the fetus, an exposure during the first trimester may produce both congenital and developmental anomalies. Later exposures are more likely to result in developmental anomalies and growth retardation. Exposure anytime during gestation may increase the likelihood of cancer.

Since the fetus may be especially sensitive to radiation, methods of preventing or reducing fetal irradiation are of interest. The simplest approach is to avoid irradiating the fetus. In many institutions, this is a very workable approach. When considering an abdominal exposure of a potentially pregnant woman, the physician should always inquire whether the patient might be pregnant. Knowledge of a pregnancy might very well alter the type of procedure being done. Whether requested or not, the patient should offer information regarding a possible pregnancy. Formal protocols (e.g., 10–14-day rule, elective booking) have been proposed to avoid fetal irradiation, but the most workable approach seems to be a direct question regarding pregnancy to women of childbearing age.[8]

If pregnancy can be ruled out, then the study can proceed as usual, with appropriate considerations for patient protection. If there is a possible or established pregnancy, some further considerations should be made. If the procedure does not constitute an emergency, it might be postponed until pregnancy is confirmed, and perhaps even delayed until after delivery, or at least until a period of greater fetal resistance to radiation. In an emergency situation, the mother's health takes precedence over that of the fetus. Hence, any necessary procedure should be done even if it involves fetal exposure. In such situations some precautions should be taken to ease the impact of the radiation on the fetus. Often some form of shielding can be used to protect the fetus. Shielding should not be used, however, if it compromises the information gained from the study, as this might render the entire radiation risk without benefit. The number of films "routinely" taken may be reduced somewhat, with a resultant decrease in patient and fetal exposure. Always, knowledge of the existence of the pregnancy, along with cooperation of the patient's physician and the radiologist, can provide significant protection of the fetus in the event of necessary exposure.

A question often raised regarding radiation and the fetus is that of termination of a pregnancy after in utero irradiation. In 1959, Hammer-Jacobsen proposed a set of guidelines based on exposure during the first 4 months of pregnancy:[9]

- Radiation exposure of the fetus to < 1 rad does not represent an indication for therapeutic abortion.
- Fetal exposures of 1–10 rad suggest therapeutic abortion only in the presence of additional indications.
- Fetal doses > 10 rad presumably suggest that therapeutic abortion be considered.

While they should not be considered absolute, modifications of these guidelines are in use at many institutions around the world. Before such recommendations can be implemented, several pieces of information must be gathered. First, the exact time of gestation at which the radiation exposure was delivered is needed. Second, a reasonably accurate estimate of the radiation dose to the fetus is necessary. This figure is determined ideally by measurements during simulation of the exposure situation. Estimates of the fetal exposure for various radiographic procedures can be obtained from the literature or several handbooks. Third, and most important, are the so-called "patient factors," such as the age and general health of the patient and her attitude toward the pregnancy and toward abortion. After these various bits of information are gathered, a decision can be reached regarding the potential hazard to the irradiated fetus and the desirability of abortion.

In our experience with some 20–30 cases involving fetal irradiation over recent years, we have not encountered a single case in which the radiation exposure was sufficiently high to warrant therapeutic termination of the pregnancy solely on the basis of the radiation exposure.[10] Nevertheless, all efforts should continue to avoid unnecessary fetal irradiation.

In summary the fetus represents a very special situation in regard to radiation exposure, as it may be peculiarly sensitive to radiation. With appropriate considerations, however, the impact of any necessary radiation exposure can be minimized.

REFERENCES

1. Bergonie J, Tribondeau L: De quelques resultats de la radiotherapie et assai de fixation d'une technique rationelle. *CR Acad Sci* (Paris) 1906:143;983.
2. Langman J: *Medical Embryology*, ed 2. Baltimore, Williams & Wilkins, 1969.
3. Russell LB, Russell WL: An analysis of the changing radiation response of the developing mouse embryo. *J Cell Comp Physiol* 1954; 43:103–149.
4. Hoffman DA, Felton RP, Cyr WH: *Effects of Ionizing Radiation on the Developing Embryo and Fetus: A Review.* Bureau of Radiological Health, 1981.
5. Rugh R: X-ray-induced teratogenesis in the mouse and its possible significance to man. *Radiology* 1971; 99:433–443.
6. Blot WJ, Miller RW: Mental retardation following in utero exposure to the atomic bombs of Hiroshima and Nagasaki. *Radiology* 1973; 106:617–619.
7. Stewart A, Kneale G: Changes in cancer risk associated with obstetric radiography. *Lancet* 1968; 1:104–107.
8. *Procedures to Minimize Diagnostic X-Ray Exposure of the Human Embryo and Fetus.* Bureau of Radiological Health, Division of Training and Medical Applications, Rockville, Maryland, 1981.
9. Hammer-Jacobsen E: Therapeutic abortion on account of x-ray examination during pregnancy. *Danish Med Bull* 1959; 6:113–122.
10. Baker ML, Vandergrift JF, Dalrymple GV: Fetal exposure in diagnostic radiology. *Health Phys* 1979; 37:237–239.

14.

Review of Genetic Concepts

Arthur Robinson

In recent years, practitioners of medicine have become increasingly aware of the importance of genetics in the understanding of physical and mental health and in the management of disease. The last decades have witnessed unprecedented developments in genetics that have increased our understanding of the basic processes of heredity enormously. New techniques and understanding have provided insights directly applicable to medicine.

The fundamental fact of heredity may be considered the ability of living organisms to produce offspring that resemble their parents more than others. One of the basic characteristics of the human condition is the uniqueness and diversity of all individuals. This results from their genetic individuality (with the exception of identical twins) and the interaction of the genetic constitution (the genome) with the environment, which is generally unique to the individual as well. In short, the interaction of genes with the environment is what confers biologic uniqueness to all humans.

More than 100 years ago, Gregor Mendel discovered the units of heredity, each responsible for a given character and segregating independently of each other. These unitary hereditary characters, later called genes, were soon shown to be positioned in a linear array on the chromosomes.

Three to four decades ago, a new era developed in biology that permanently changed the basic nature of this science. This revolution, called molecular biology, explained many biologic properties in terms of chemistry and paved the way for the explosion of new and fundamental knowledge of genetic processes that is undergoing exponential growth all around us. During this period of increasing knowledge there also developed a realization of the major burden that genetic disease imposes on our population, thus explaining the medical profession's growing interest in genetics.

The central structure of any living cell is in the nucleus, where the genes reside on the chromosomes. The DNA of the gene has a dual function: (1) to replicate itself, a process that constitutes the central act of reproduction; and (2) to be responsible for the chemical reactions of the cell, its metabolism.

All the chemical reactions within cells require the catalytic action of spe-

131

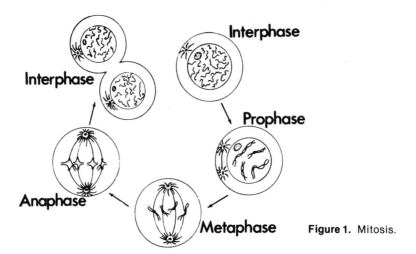

Figure 1. Mitosis.

cific proteins called enzymes, consisting of a linear array of amino acids, the nature and position of which are determined by a series of consecutive triplet base pairs in the linear DNA chain. Many of the details of how this information in the DNA is transcribed and translated have been defined, and the process has been duplicated in vitro using cell extracts. Most recent information testifies to the variety and increasing complexity of regulatory mechanisms that modify the different stages of transcription and translation. The

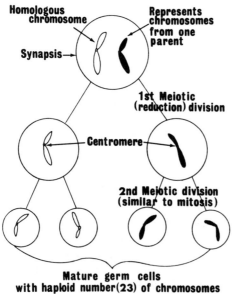

Figure 2. Meiosis.

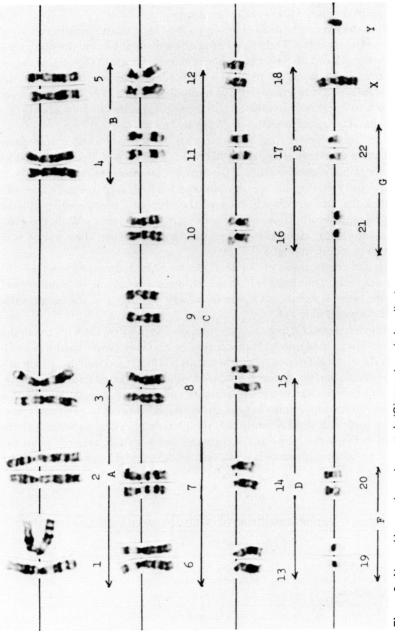

Figure 3. Normal human karyotype, male (Giemsa-trypsin banding).

techniques of recombinant DNA and restriction enzymes have made it possible to examine these operations in much greater detail, thus unraveling new universes in the clarification of the hereditary processes.[1]

Human cells can be divided into two types: the somatic (nonsex cells) and the gametes (sex cells). The former divide by a form of asexual division called mitosis (Fig. 1) and the latter (sperm and ovum) by meiosis (Fig. 2), a process that reduces the usual 23 pairs of chromosomes (diploid number) of the somatic cells to 23 chromosomes (the haploid number). When fertilization of the ovum by sperm occurs, the fertilized egg regains the 23 pairs of chromosomes characteristic of human somatic cells.

The first documentation of the fact that the normal human chromosome complement (karyotype) contained 46 chromosomes was in 1956,[2] followed by the first complete identification of the human chromosomes by Tjio and Puck in 1958.[3] In 1959, the Human Chromosome Study Group[4] met in Denver and produced the Denver Classification of the Human Chromosomes, still the basis of the universally agreed-upon system of nomenclature. With new cytogenetic knowledge, especially the new banding techniques, the system was to some extent modified (Fig. 3).[5]

An unforeseen result of the development of human cytogenetics was the realization that abnormalities of the chromosomes, both in number and structure, were a significant cause of human wastage and serious developmental disease (Table 1).[6]

Newer cytogenetic techniques, especially the most recent high-resolution methods,[7] have made possible much greater resolving power than was available in the original Denver classification. In addition to identifying many new chromosomal diseases, these techniques have demonstrated an interesting relationship between karyotypic abnormalities and malignancy. Although it has been known for some time that the chromosomal content of most malignant tissue is disturbed, until recently only the Philadelphia chromosome, a translocation between the long arms of chromosomes 9 and 22, has been related to a specific malignancy, namely, chronic myelogenous leukemia (Fig. 4). With

TABLE 1. INCIDENCE OF GROSS CHROMOSOMAL ABNORMALITIES*

Group	%
All conceptions	5–10
Spontaneous abortions (first and second trimester)	30–50
Live births	0.5

*The new staining techniques have revealed that minor abnormalities are commoner than previously thought.

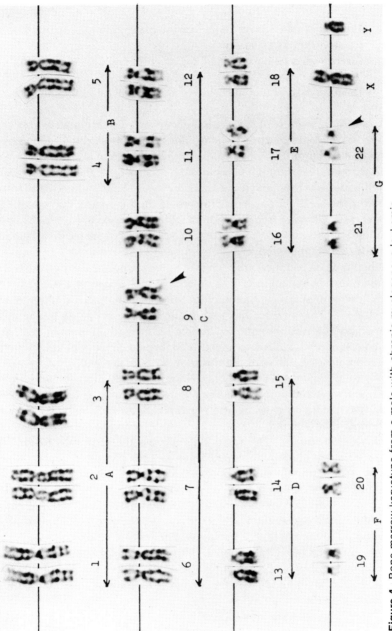

Figure 4. Bone marrow karyotype from a male with chronic myelogenous leukemia showing the Philadelphia chromosome [t(9q;22q)].

the ability to look at chromosomal anatomy in greater detail, the following associations have also been made:

1. Interstitial deletion on short arm of chromosome 11 (p13): Wilms' tumor aniridia syndrome
2. Interstitial deletion on long arm of chromosome 13 (q24): Retinoblastoma
3. Deletion in short arm of chromosome 3: Small cell carcinoma of lung

In addition, a group of four recessively inherited conditions — xeroderma pigmentosa, Bloom's dwarfism, congenital aplastic anemia, and ataxia telangiectasia — all of which predispose to the production of cancer, are now called chromosomal instability syndromes because of the increased susceptibility of their chromosomes to breakage by exogenous physical or chemical factors, or both. Of particular interest is the suggestion that carriers of these genes (much more frequent than the affected persons) may also be sensitive to these agents and may represent subpopulations of people with a greater likelihood of developing cancer.[8]

An important technical advance made possible by our current abilities to culture and study human cells in vitro (somatic cell genetics) is the ability to localize genes to specific chromosomes, and even to specific parts of the chromosomes. This advance has been made possible primarily by the technique of interspecific somatic cell fusion. A mixture of human cells and rodent cells, when exposed to inactivated Sendai virus, will result in the production of fused cells with the chromosome complements of both species. In order to identify these so-called heterokaryons, the cells from both species usually possess a mutation, so that the rodent cell (mouse or Chinese hamster ovary, CHO) cannot grow by itself in a medium deficient in a specific metabolite. The human cell is in a similar situation, except that the metabolite is different. The fused cells will be the only cells to grow in medium deficient in both substances, since they can complement each other's needs by synthesizing the substance that the other cell cannot make by reason of its mutation. When these cells are grown continuously in the doubly deficient medium, the human chromosomes are sequentially lost, with the exception of the chromosome that has on it the gene responsible for complementing the mutation in the CHO cell. In this way, genes can be localized to specific chromosomes and even to parts of chromosomes, since the only human chromosomal material left in the fused cell must have the gene for the essential substance. Some 300–350 human genes have by now been localized in the human genome.[9]

Once the genes have been located, it may become possible, by the techniques of molecular biology and recombinant DNA, to identify the errors in the DNA associated with mutations; in short, to recognize a mutation by looking at the DNA itself (present in all cells) rather than at the product, a protein, in certain specialized tissues only. As a result, these techniques will undoubtedly greatly influence our ability to understand the molecular basis of many genetic diseases, with all that implies for prevention, early diagnosis, and treatment.

Medical genetics today is the application to the practice of medicine of all the new insights we have briefly touched on. Simultaneously with these new insights, and to some degree because of them, has come the realization of the great burden on society and the untold suffering caused by diseases that are genetic in origin.[10-12] Some of this impact is listed as follows:

1. Thirty to 50 percent of spontaneous abortions are associated with chromosomal malformations.
2. Eight to 10 percent of stillbirths are associated with chromosomal malformations.
3. One of 150 live births is associated with chromosomal malformations.
4. Three percent of live births have other genetic diseases, including congenital malformations.
5. Twenty percent of patients in childrens' hospitals have diseases primarily genetic in origin.
6. Twenty-five percent of those with chronic diseases, or approximately 12×10^6 people in the United States, have a genetic disorder. Total years of life lost from birth defects are 3.5 times greater than for cancer, 6.5 times greater than for heart disease, and 8 times greater than for stroke.

As a result of the frequency of genetic disorders and their potential for prevention, medical genetics is also entering the domain of public health. Medical genetics can in fact be considered a form of preventive medicine.

Three varieties of clinical genetic practice will be briefly discussed: preconceptional and postconceptional genetic counseling and genetic screening.

Genetic counseling, a major part of the practice of medical genetics, concerns itself with giving couples information from which they can make responsible and informed decisions about reproduction—something only the human member of the animal kingdom is capable of doing.

Preconceptional genetic counseling is usually sought by couples who fear that some condition that has previously appeared in their families might recur should they reproduce. The counselor must confirm the correct diagnosis, determine whether the condition is hereditary, and, if so, evaluate what kind of inheritance is operative. The counseling of the patients then centers around the odds and stakes involved, the former being a statistical consideration, and the latter being a subjective appraisal of the burden of the condition should it recur. The counselor also presents various alternatives, namely, adopt, wait, take a chance, undergo amniocentesis (see below), or opt for artificial insemination by donor (AID), depending on which approach is genetically appropriate.

Postconceptional genetic counseling has had its major development during the past 10 years. The question to be answered for pregnant women before the advent of genetic amniocentesis was: Are the odds and stakes sufficient to constitute a valid indication for interrupting the pregnancy? For most cases, the final decision was based on the patient's evaluation of the probabilities. A low statistical risk (<3 percent) could often be more than a person could face, if the burden in her mind was very high.

In contrast, genetic amniocentesis has in many cases changed the probability of a fetus being affected or unaffected to a certainty. The procedure consists of introducing a needle into the uterus at about 15 weeks' gestation and removing some of the fluid in which the fetus is bathed. Fetal cells in the fluid can then be grown by the techniques of somatic cell genetics, so that indicated chromosomal or biochemical assays can be performed. Some of the newer techniques mentioned earlier promise to increase vastly our ability to diagnose fetal disease. In addition, our increased familiarity with the fetus and its intrauterine environment is making possible a new branch of medicine, fetal medicine, including possibilities of gene repair and surgical correction of progressive fetal malformations, such as hydrocephalus, in utero.[13]

Another aspect of genetic preventive medicine is genetic screening of various populations. In general use at this time is the screening of newborns for a variety of serious metabolic conditions, so that early diagnosis and treatment can be instituted before the onset of serious and irreversible symptoms that, if not lethal, will inevitably produce mental retardation. These conditions include phenylketonuria, galactosemia, congenital hypothyroidism, and maple syrup urine disease, all serious neonatal diseases requiring early diagnosis and treatment.

The other type of genetic screening includes identification of subpopulations of persons who, by virtue of their genetic makeup, are at increased risk to produce defective offspring. These are people who may require specific environmental manipulations to counteract their specific susceptibilities (such as susceptibility to emphysema associated with alpha-1-antitrypsin deficiency or susceptibility to coronary disease associated with familial hyperlipoproteinemia). Another group consists of persons who carry a recessive mutant gene but who are normal. When one of the latter mates with a similar carrier, there is a 1:4 chance that the resulting offspring will have the same mutant gene on both of the homologous chromosomes (homozygote) and will evidence serious disease (Tay-Sachs disease in Jews of Eastern European origin, sickle cell anemia in blacks).

Subjects of further discussion would include artificial insemination by

donor, an excellent genetic solution of many problems; fetoscopy, an important advance in intrauterine diagnosis; and in vitro fertilization as a relief to
thousands of women with certain kinds of infertility. These techniques pose
ethical and social problems that society is just beginning to consider.

REFERENCES

1. Emery AEH: Recombinant DNA technology. *Lancet* 1981; 2:1406-1409.
2. Tjio JH, Levan A: The chromosome number of man. *Hereditas* 1956; 42:1-6.
3. Tjio JH, Puck TT: The somatic chromosomes of man. *Proc Natl Acad Sci USA* 1958; 44:1229-1237.
4. The Human Chromosome Study Group (14 signatories): A proposed standard system of nomenclature of human mitotic chromosomes. *Am J Hum Genet* 1960; 12:384-388.
5. Caspersson T, Zech L, Johansson C, et al: Identification of human chromosomes by DNA binding fluorescent agents. *Chromosoma* 1970; 30:215-227.
6. Warburton D: Current techniques in chromosome analysis. *Pediatr Clin North Am* 1980; 27:753-767.
7. Yunis JJ, Sanchez O: The G-banded prophase chromosomes of man. *Humangenetik* 1975; 27:167-172.
8. Swift M: Malignant neoplasms in heterozygous carriers of genes for certain auto-somal recessive syndromes. In Mulvihill JJ, Miller RW, Fraumeni JF (eds): *Genetics of Human Cancer. Progress in Cancer Research and Therapy*, vol 3. New York, Raven Press, 1977; pp 209-215.
9. Kao FT, Johnson RT, Puck TT: Complementation analysis on virus-fused Chinese hamster cells with nutritional markers. *Science* 1969, 164:312-314.
10. Desforges JF: Current concepts in genetics. Editorial *N Engl J Med* 1976; 294:393.
11. Trimble BK, Doughty JH: The amount of hereditary disease in human popula-tions. *Ann Hum Genet* 1974; 38:199-223.
12. Day N, Holmes LB: The incidence of genetic disease in a university hospital population. *Am J Hum Genet* 1973; 25:237-246.
13. Clewell WH, Johnson ML, Meier PR, et al: A surgical approach to the treat-ment of fetal hydrocephalus. *N Engl J Med* 1982; 306:1320-1325.

15.

Genetic Consequences of Radiation Exposure

Arthur Robinson

Genetic effects, referring as they do to effects on future generations, are among the most elusive and also the most controversial of the health effects of exposure to radiation. This discussion relies heavily on the report of the Committee on the Biological Effects of Ionizing Radiations (BEIR-III).[1]

In 1927, Muller exposed fruit flies to x-rays and was able to show for the first time that ionizing radiation increases the frequency of mutations, sudden permanent changes in DNA.[2] The site of mutation is randomly determined, hence repeated doses to the germ cells will not produce the same result each time. It has since become clear that radiations penetrating the human gonadal cells are genetically undesirable because of the production of mutations in the germ cells. Other mutagenic agents are heat, chemicals, and viruses.

We now know that both gene mutations and chromosomal aberrations are produced by ionizing radiation. A gene mutation is produced when a nucleotide in the DNA molecule is changed so that an altered triplet sequence of base pairs will code for a different amino acid. One example of such a mutation is conversion of the sixth amino acid in the β-polypeptide chain of hemoglobin A from glutamic acid to valine. The resultant mutant protein is sickle cell hemoglobin, the basis for sickle cell anemia. Other mutations having even more serious effects are so-called frame-shift mutants in which the addition or deletion of a nucleotide in the DNA shifts the reading sequence of the code. This shift can change whole sequences of amino acids in the protein until the defect is corrected for by a reverse shift.

A germ cell with a mutation does not pass to the fertilized egg the particular parental trait involved; instead, it produces an altered, defective trait that would "breed true" in future generations.

The expression "genetic hazards of radiation" refers to the danger of radiation to future generations. This expression distinguishes genetic hazards from the somatic effects of radiation, which may also be associated with

141

damage to genetic material (i.e., damage to the chromosomes of somatic cells). In the latter situation, the effects are limited to the person exposed to the radiation and not to descendants of the person. Unfortunately, there is almost a complete absence of information on radiation-induced mutations in humans, especially at low levels of exposure. What little information we do have is based on laboratory animal data, with the attendant risks of extrapolating from mouse to humans and of having to hypothesize the most probable genetic effects of low doses from those at relatively high doses. We do know, however, through the techniques of somatic cell genetics, that human somatic cells are at least as sensitive to reproductive killing by radiation as those of any other animals, lending some credibility to the extrapolation.[3]

So-called "spontaneous" mutations occur all the time from a variety of causes, mostly unknown. Only a small percentage of them (about 6 percent) is caused by background radiation.[1] It has been estimated that one out of five people has a new "spontaneous" mutation that his or her parents did not have, and that the average person carries a genetic load of about eight undesirable genes.[4] Moreover, the mutation induced by ionizing radiation is qualitatively no different from a spontaneous mutation. It is not unique. Consequently, it is difficult to study the genetic effects of radiation, because they can be measured only by quantitatively identifying an increase in the expected rate of mutations.

A few generalizations can safely be made[1]:

1. Most mutations are undesirable, although some are apparently indifferent.
2. Radiation increases the probability of a mutation.
3. The effects of radiation-induced mutations are no different from those of "spontaneous" mutations.
4. The mutagenic effects of radiation are probably cumulative.
5. There is no evidence that there is a dose below which there is no mutagenic effect, although there is controversy about whether straight-line proportionality persists down to the very lowest doses.

Currently, the only way to judge the mutagenic effect of radiation in humans is to count the increase in heritable defects in an irradiated population. These effects are caused by damage to (1) a single gene, (2) a chromosome in which the damage might affect many genes, or (3) a so-called indeterminate effect. The latter is a more complex type of genetic effect that can generally be described as a gene mutation of minor effect capable of producing changes in susceptibility and of influencing every aspect of our mental, as well as physical, well-being.[1]

An increase in mutations will increase the frequency of certain conditions, but at markedly different rates, depending on the nature of the inheritance of the trait affected. Recessive mutations are the most common form of mutations. In recessive mutations, the mutated gene must be present on both members of a pair of homologous chromosomes (the homozygous condition) for the mutation to be expressed as a disease such as phenylketonuria. This expression may not occur for many generations, depending on when two carriers for the same mutated gene happen to mate. On the other hand, a change in the mutation rate of an autosomal dominantly inherited condition such as Huntington's chorea, in which the trait will reveal itself when the mutation is on only one of a pair of chromosomes (in the heterozygote), will increase the incidence of the condition rapidly (in one or two generations).

The male, with only one X chromosome, will express recessive mutations located on a single X. Hence, diseases such as muscular dystrophy and hemophilia, both sex-linked recessively inherited traits, occur primarily in the male. These mutations are somewhat similar to dominant mutations located on other chromosomes (autosomes) because they are usually expressed within a few generations, as opposed to many generations later, as happens with recessive mutations.

As mentioned before, radiation can also produce chromosomal damage, such as an alteration in chromosome number or structure. In general, aberrations of chromosome number are not frequently caused by low doses of radiation. When they occur, they probably prevent a viable birth, or even a recognizable pregnancy. The occurrence of Down's syndrome, caused by the presence of an extra chromosome 21, has in some studies been related to relatively low radiation exposures.[5-7] Other studies have not confirmed this relationship.[8-10] Ionizing radiation is more likely to produce chromosomal imbalances, by causing breakage and rearrangement of chromosomes or loss of small segments of chromosomes.

Finally, there is another class of mutation in *Drosophila* the effects of which are so mild that they can be detected only by exposing large numbers of fruit flies. These are the most frequent class of radiation-induced mutations in *Drosophila* and are also more frequent in mice. In humans, these mutations could produce polygenic effects that might be responsible for greater susceptibility to disease.

Because of the heterogeneity in the nature and timing of mutational effects produced by radiation (or other mutagens), and because of the complicating factors resulting from the occurrence of similar conditions arising from other causes, radiation might have important effects on human well-being, yet still go unnoticed.

The gene pool (i.e., the total number of genes in the population) defines the incidence of genetic mutations and therefore the extent of genetic disease in the population. From the perspective of the gene pool, it is evident that small doses of radiation to a large population are genetically more undesirable than large doses to a small population, since in the former case there would be a greater dilution of the gene pool with undesirable mutants. As a result, the focus of concern today in advisory and regulatory agencies is the effect of low doses on the population as a whole and the need to control the overall population dose.

The National Academy of Sciences Committee on the Biological Effects of Ionizing Radiations (BEIR-III) has stressed that exposure to radiation from sources other than background should be kept as low as possible, since any dose might have potential for genetic harm. Currently, the estimated radiation to the average U.S. citizen during the reproductive years is thought to be 3 rem from background, 1.5 rem from medical sources, and 0.3 rem from a variety of environmental sources. Hence, background supplies the major natural contribution and medical exposure the major nonbackground induced contribution.[1]

It must be stressed that these recommendations are little more than educated guesses, since there is no unequivocal evidence of radiation-induced mutants in humans, although they have been produced in human cells in vitro.[3]

To study the expected effects of radiation in comparison to the current incidence of genetic effects, the concept of the doubling dose is used. The doubling dose is the genetically effective radiation dose that would induce as many mutations per generation as arise spontaneously. This concept can be employed to estimate the increased risk of general disease attributable to increased radiation exposure to a population. The doubling dose for humans has been estimated at 20–200 rem by extrapolating from studies on *Drosophila* and on mice, as well as from A-bomb data from Japan. A doubling dose of 40 rem might increase the number of mutant genes per person from 8.0 to 8.2 and would be hard to detect. It has been estimated that if one considers the doubling dose for humans to be 20–200 rem in the United States, an additional dose of 5 rem would produce 100–1800 cases of serious dominant and X-linked diseases in the first generation. Currently, we know of about 1000 gene defects that affect about 1 percent of the newborn population.

In conclusion, the following statements seem appropriate:

1.   The benefits of radiation are seen immediately. The somatic hazards are to the person exposed. The genetic hazards are remote and affect persons in future generations.
2.   The average exposure to the population should be less than that permitted for individuals. It is the average dose to the gene pool that determines mutation rates to the population.
3.   Radiation-induced mutations are not unique, hence are hard to recognize. The mutagenic effect is an increase in the probability that

some unidentified person born generations from now will have a defect.

4. It is the total and chronic exposure from conception to the end of the reproductive period that has a genetic significance.

5. Medical radiation is still the major nonbackground contributor to genetic risk. Its use should be limited to appropriately trained and qualified persons. Certainly, no exposure should be permitted without expectation of commensurate benefit.

REFERENCES

1. BEIR-III: *The Effects on Populations of Exposure to Low Levels of Ionizing Radiation: 1980.* Washington DC, Committee on the Biological Effects of Ionizing Radiations. National Academy Press, 1980.

2. Muller HJ: Artificial transmutation of the gene. *Science* 1927; 66:84–87.

3. Puck TT, Marcus P: Action of x-rays on mammalian cells. *J Exp Med* 1956; 103:653.

4. Russell WL: Radiation in mice; the genetic effects and their implications for man. *Bull Atom Sci* 1956; 12:19.

5. Alberman E, Polani PE, Roberts JAF, et al: Parental exposures to x-irradiation and Down's syndrome. *Ann Hum Genet* 1972; 36:195–208.

6. Cohen BH, Lilienfeld AM: The epidemiological study of mongolism in Baltimore. *Ann NY Acad Sci* 1970; 171:320–327.

7. Uchida I, Curtis EJ: A possible association between maternal radiation and mongolism. *Lancet* 1961; 2:848.

8. Lunn JE: A survey of mongol children in Glasgow. *Scott Med J* 1959; 4:368–372.

9. Schull WJ, Neel JV: Maternal radiation and mongolism. *Lancet* 1962; 1:537–538.

10. Carter CO, Evans KA, Stewart AM: Maternal irradiation and Down's syndrome (mongolism). *Lancet* 1961; 2:1042.

16.

Protection in Diagnostic Radiology: Historic Perspectives

Glenn V. Dalrymple
Max L. Baker

In the first radiograph of a human ever made, W.C. Roentgen applied what was to become a basic principle of radiation protection. He exposed, as best he could, only his patient—in this case his wife. He did not expose himself to the radiation beam. For this historic radiograph, Roentgen used a photographic plate exposed for approximately 15 minutes. Almost from the beginning, a few investigators recognized the potentially detrimental effects of these "new kinds of rays." These early workers, observing the skin changes with the long exposure times and soft radiation of the old gas tubes, began to make some efforts at both patient and physician protection. Further development of the field of radiology showed improvements in both equipment and film, as well as parallel improvement in protection procedures.

The initial radiographic picture used a photographic emulsion on a glass plate. By 1920, however, this type of plate was becoming a rarity. World War I made the acquisition of glass plates difficult, and for several years film had been used increasingly as a support for the photographic emulsion. In 1914 Eastman Kodak introduced large (11 × 17-inch) single coated film with a radiation sensitivity greater than any available plate.

Film was clearly superior to plates in most respects. Not only was film more sensitive to radiation, which meant lower radiation doses to the patient, it also was less fragile and thus easier to handle and store. One disadvantage of this film, however, was the flammability of the cellulose nitrate base. (For example, in 1929 a film fire started by cellulose nitrate film claimed 124 lives at a Cleveland clinic.) Thereafter, cellulose acetate became the film base and remained in use for many years. Today most films have a polyester base. With these improved films and progress in development chemistry, the radiation dose to the patient was lowered by as much as 75 percent.

Introduction of the intensifying screen further reduced the dose to the patient. This device consists of a thin layer of tiny phosphor crystals coated onto a cardboard or plastic support. Each crystal absorbs x-ray energy and emits an amount of light directly related to the amount of x-ray energy absorbed. Over the surface of the screen, differences in x-ray intensity are transformed into differences in light intensity to which the film is highly sensitive. The entire image is thus "intensified" for recording by the film. This concept, originally suggested by Dr. William Herbert Rollins of Boston in 1902, was in common use by World War II.[1]

After the war, improvements in screens lowered the patient exposure by as much as 50 percent over previous techniques. In recent years, the introduction of "rare earth" intensifying screens has resulted in another 50 percent or so reduction in patient dose.

Beam collimation devices have also significantly reduced the population exposure from medical radiation. These devices limit the field of x-ray exposure to the area of film, so that no unnecessary tissue is irradiated. The idea of this device we also owe to the genius of Dr. William Herbert Rollins, who, in 1901 suggested that "No x-light should strike a patient except the smallest beam that will cover the area to be examined, photographed, or treated."[2]

While the idea of the collimator, and indeed its common use in the x-ray facility, is quite old, laws requiring such devices on x-ray machines came into being only as a part of the Radiation Control for Health and Safety Act of 1968.[3] This brings up an important concept in the development of radiation protection standards. At least in the health professions, radiation protection has progressed largely as a voluntary effort. While many of the regulations and recommendations are now a matter of law, they were developed and applied for many years voluntarily by most radiation users before passage of the law. As equipment has improved and knowledge of radiation effects has increased, radiation protection measures have improved largely as a voluntary effort.

Whereas all the previously described techniques have served to lower patient radiation doses, and indeed many diagnostic radiographic procedures are associated with relatively low doses, there is still the potential to receive higher doses than necessary from many procedures. The more common procedures such as x-ray films of the chest expose the patient to radiation levels similar to that of natural background. As the complexity of the procedure increases, however, the patient dose generally increases as well. The addition of extensive fluroroscopy to an x-ray procedure, such as in arteriography or cardiac catheterization, adds especially to the total patient exposure.

Thus, while radiation protection measures have significantly lowered the radiation dose to the patient and the worker, there comes a point beyond which further reductions might not be feasible, either from an economic or technical standpoint. Even these low levels of radiation carry an associated risk. What then are some of the health hazards associated with radiation exposure?

According to the "nonthreshold" model of radiation injury, any radiation exposure carries with it a finite probability of biologic damage.[4] This damage might be in the form of an increased risk of cancer induction or subsequent cancer death, or possibly genetic damage. The nonthreshold model presupposes an increase in these biological risks with every increment of radiation exposure.

The biologic effects of radiation have been under study almost from the time of the discovery of x-rays and radioactivity. The first injuries to humans were described early in 1896, and the first death attributed to x-rays was that of Thomas Edison's assistant, Clarence Dally in 1904.[5] These effects were of considerable interest and concern during the early part of the twentieth century, and a number of standards were developed to protect the workers and patients from the effects of radiation. During the Manhattan Project (the code name for the U.S. effort to develop an atomic bomb during World War II), a great deal of interest was focused upon the potential biological effects of atomic radiation. Since that time there has been a progressively increasing interest in the biologic effects of radiation, with the development of a separate science (radiation biology), and a number of scientific societies (e.g., Radiation Research Society, Health Physics Society) devoted to the field of radiation effects and radiation protection.

While the various models of biologic injury indicate that, in a population sense, there may be a small hazard from radiation, the risk to any specific individual in the population is extremely small. In part because of the unobjective coverage of radiation related events in the news media, many people have developed a fear about the potential impact of any exposure to radiation. Consequently, patients increasingly question their physicians regarding the benefits as well as the risks of diagnostic procedures that use radiation.

One of the most difficult questions to answer is: What is a necessary x-ray examination? Perhaps an appropriate answer is: An examination is necessary if the patient's treatment will be compromised without it. In many clinical situations, however, there are few or no clear-cut criteria for a given study. The physician must then make a decision regarding the use of x-ray studies on the basis of professional experience and uncertainty about the patient's condition at the time. Unfortunately, the physician's decision may also be tempered by personal sensitivity to the standards of practice in his or her community, and especially by fear of malpractice litigation if the study is not performed. These types of issues lead to the question: How often are unnecessary x-ray examinations performed? While this question is probably unanswerable, there is no question but that unnecessary examinations, for whatever reason, do increase the health care costs and radiation exposure to the public.

Besides the question of unnecessary x-ray studies, there is a problem of irradiation of parts of the body outside the area of interest. In the past, x-ray equipment frequently permitted the exposure of large volumes of tissue that were not imaged on the film. Under current guidelines, the radiation beam must be limited by machine design to the size of the image receptor. These automatic devices may be bypassed by the operator, however, and should not be considered absolute in function. In addition to automatic collimation, gonadal shielding is a form of protection to the patient. A variety of gonadal shields for males are available; one type or another should be used when the gonads are in or near the direct beam. Gonadal shields for females are technically more difficult to design, but are under development. Use of the shields does not compromise the information needed for diagnosis.

Another important problem related to radiation protection is that of poor-quality radiography. All x-ray examinations should be performed by properly trained and registered technologists. These technologists should be supervised by a physician trained in the technical aspects of radiology and in the interpretation of the x-ray films. The x-ray equipment should be in good condition, properly maintained, and used with high-quality x-ray film, intensifying screens, and proper film processing. Unfortunately, x-ray procedures are performed in circumstances in which these criteria are not always met. For example, although 70 percent of all radiographs are supervised by a trained radiologist, a sizable portion of these studies are performed by non-registered technologists. Some states now require minimal educational standards for x-ray personnel, and recent congressional action probably will result in additional states following this action.

Within the context of health hazards, the question of the pregnant or potentially pregnant patient has previously been considered at some length. As indicated earlier, any x-ray examination that is not indicated by the patient's condition should be avoided. If the study is indicated and pregnancy cannot be ruled out, a limited study (i.e., a reduced number of films) should be conducted whenever possible. Obviously when the patient's life and health are in jeopardy, radiation effects on the fetus are secondary to the welfare of the mother (see Chapter 13).

The biologic effects, both real and potential, of ionizing radiation are related to the distribution of the radiation in tissue. Generally, the effect is reduced if a smaller volume of tissue is irradiated. With radioisotopes used in nuclear medicine, the relative tissue distribution of the isotope determines the distribution of radiation dose and consequently the potential biologic effect. For example, technetium pertechnetate used in thyroid scanning is secreted by the salivary glands, the gastric mucosa, and to a lesser extent the kidneys. A significant amount of this isotope stays within the gastrointestinal (GI) tract, delivering the greatest radiation dose to the colon. In contrast, almost all the technetium-labeled diethylenetriaminepentaacetic acid (DTPA) used in brain scanning is eliminated through the kidneys, ureters, and bladder, and these structures receive the highest radiation dose. Thus, different chemical forms of the same radioisotope deliver their greatest radiation doses to different areas. Other radioisotopes are also localized in specific organs. For example, iodine-131 is accumulated by the thyroid and iron-59 by the bone marrow. Because of these differences in the biologic distribution of the radioisotope and the wide range of associated types and energies of radiation, a separate dosimetry approach has been developed for medically administered radioisotopes.[6] This approach permits calculation of radiation doses based on the kinetics of the biologic systems involved as well as on the physical characteristics of the radiation. For all practical purposes, radiation doses from nuclear medicine studies are of the same order of magnitude as those from diagnostic x-ray examinations. Doses to specific organs, however, may be quite different.

One of the newer imaging modalities, computed tomographic (CT) scanning is in some ways a variation of a conventional diagnostic x-ray study. In CT a conventional x-ray tube serves as the radiation source, but a series of electronic radiation detectors rather than film is used to measure the transmission of x-rays through the patient. This transmission information is gathered and processed by a computer. The physician can visualize very subtle changes in patient anatomy, while keeping patient exposure to a reasonable level.

When examining radiation protection from the historic perspective, current radiation protection guidelines for maximum permissible doses (MPD) for radiation workers are of interest. In 1931, the MPD was 50 rem/year. Since that time, the MPD has been revised downward three times to its present level of 5 rem/year. This reduction by a factor of 10 resulted more from an ability to use radiation in an increasingly safe manner than from an increased knowledge of radiation effects, although this factor certainly contributed to the reduction. Present considerations suggest that a concept entitled ALARA (*As Low As Reasonably Achievable*) should be instituted in addition to the 5-rem/year value.[7] It is hoped that this addition would serve to decrease the population exposure further by removing the impression that an "acceptable" maximum for radiation exposure exists.

In conclusion, to the question: Can we get rid of ionizing radiation in medicine? the answer is probably: In all probability, no. Diagnostic radiation is here to stay, at least for the foreseeable future. Newer diagnostic modalities using x-rays are being developed that, aided by computers and other electronic improvements, may well continue to lower patient and population exposures to radiation.

In addition, imaging techniques with nonionizing radiation are being increasingly used in radiology. Ultrasound, for example, employs very high frequency sound waves in the place of ionizing radiation. There is some question about the absolute safety of ultrasound. On a theoretical basis, however, there is little support for potential biologic damage from ultrasound, at least as compared with x-rays.[8] Nuclear magnetic resonance is another new imaging technique. While the effect of strong magnetic fields on biologic systems is unknown, initial experiments have shown no detectable harm.[9] Medical thermography is also enjoying renewed interest, particularly in the areas of pain management and vascular disorders.

No exposure to ionizing radiation is without risk. In the hands of a skilled user, however, the risk:benefit ratio appears to be highly skewed toward the benefit side for both the patient and the physician.

REFERENCES

1. Brecher R, Brecher E: *The Rays*. Baltimore, Williams & Wilkins, 1969; p 426.
2. Rollins W: *Notes on X-Light*. Boston, privately published, 1904; pp 260-272.
3. Radiation Control for Health and Safety Act of 1968.
4. BEIR-III: *The Effects on Populations of Exposure to Low Levels of Ionizing Radiation*. Washington DC, Committee of the Biological Effects of Ionizing Radiation, National Academy Press, 1980.
5. Brown P: *American Martyrs to Science through the Roentgen Rays*. Springfield, Ill, Charles C Thomas, 1936.
6. MIRD: *MIRD Pamphlets*. Medical Internal Radiation Dose Committee, Society of Nuclear Medicine, New York, NY.
7. ICRP: *Recommendations of the International Commission in Radiological Protection*. ICRP Report 26. Oxford, Pergamon, 1977.
8. Baker ML, Dalrymple GV: Biological effects of diagnostic ultrasound: A review. *Radiology* 1978; 126:479-483.
9. Wolff S, Crooks LE, Brown P, et al: Tests for DNA and chromosomal damage induced by nuclear magnetic resonance imaging. *Radiology* 1980; 136:707-710.

17.

History of Radiation Protection Agencies and Standards

E. Russell Ritenour

When W.C. Roentgen discovered x-rays in 1895 there was little reason to regard them as dangerous. After all, the light from the sun was not particularly dangerous unless one was exposed to it for a long time. Even then, reddening of the skin would occur and the exposure could be terminated. It required no great judgment to determine that overexposure to the sun's rays caused sunburn a few hours later. When demonstrable physiologic changes did not occur soon after exposure to x-rays, many early experiments deemed them safe, even beneficial. Others, however, began to suspect that reported ulcerations, swelling, and scarring of the hands, although occurring some time after exposure, were indeed caused by exposure to the new ray.

The earliest reports of symptoms (eye irritation) after exposure to x-rays were reported independently by Edison, Morton, and Tesla in March 1896.[1] Ironically, these reports were probably in error. It is likely that the sensations were caused by eye strain or ultraviolet from the fluorescence and not from the x-rays themselves. Nevertheless, reports of adverse skin effects were becoming more frequent. In late 1896 Thomson purposely exposed the little finger of his left hand (intermittently) to an x-ray tube for several days.[2] This unusually large exposure brought immediate effects, and he chronicled the symptoms of pain, swelling, and stiffness as they appeared. Here was rather convincing evidence of a causal link between exposure to x-rays and adverse health effects.

Still, many argued that x-rays were harmless in all but the most extreme cases. Some held this opinion because they realized that the public's fascination with the mysterious new rays could be exploited for financial gain. By the turn of the century, most physicians and scientists who were knowledgeable in this field were aware, at least qualitatively, of the hazards. In 1902 one of Thomas Edison's assistants who tested x-ray tubes during their manufacture developed skin cancer and died. His death was reasonably attributed to his occupational exposure.[2]

There was at least one early advocate of radiation protection. William Herbert Rollins, a Boston dentist, made many fundamental contributions to safety during the first years of this century. Among these were lead shielding, collimators, and higher-voltage x-ray tubes to decrease the unnecessary low-energy x-rays absorbed in the patient.[3] However, the first formal statement of radiation protection by a professional society was not made until 1913.[4] The German Roentgen Ray Society released a report that included a specific recommendation of 2 mm lead shielding to protect operators of x-ray equipment from leakage radiation. Two years later, the British Roentgen Society made some general statements concerning the need for formulation of safety regulations.[5] Unfortunately, World War I intervened, and for several years safety standards were considered an unnecessary luxury.

Interest in radiation protection revived in 1920 when news articles appeared concerning the leukemic deaths of five workers and a prominent x-ray physician at the London Radium Institute.[4] The result was the formation of the British Xray and Radium Protection Committee. The French Academy of Medicine soon followed with a special study commission. The British and French made similar recommendations having to do with shielding, working hours, blood examinations for workers, and so on.

As reflected in the British and French recommendations, the assumption at this time was that an amount of radiation exists below which there are no ill effects and above which a danger is present. By 1925 at least four researchers had independently arrived at essentially the same value for this "tolerance dose."[5] Each translated the tolerance dose as roughly one-hundredth of the amount of radiation required to produce erythema (redness of the skin). This amount was not to be exceeded within 1 month's time. The erythema dose was not well quantified, and we know today that it depends on many factors, such as the area of the body exposed, the energy of the beam, an individual's sensitivity to radiation, and so on. By 1927, it was known that the value of the erythema dose varied from 100 to 700 R. However, researchers were not yet in agreement as to the precise definition of the roentgen.[5] One-hundredth of an erythema dose per month was chosen because it represented the amount of radiation below which no harm had been seen at the various research and clinical institutions. In addition, another factor of 10 or so had been included for safety's sake. These early attempts laid the foundation of modern protection standards. As observed by Taylor in a 1978 symposium on the history of radiation protection standards, what we have today is "a large array of philosophy built on observing nothing."[5]

The same year that the tolerance dose was defined, the first meeting of the International Congress of Radiology was held in London.[5] At this meeting a study group, The International Commission on Radiation Units and Measurements (ICRU), was formed to look into the standardization of the measurement of radiation. At the Second International Congress in Stockholm in 1928, the "roentgen" was adopted as the official unit of x-ray measurement.[6] A quantification of protection standards was now possible, and the Second Congress formed a seven-member International Commission on X-ray and Radium Protection, later known as the International Commission on Radiological Protection (ICRP) to investigate this quantification.[5] Some interim protection recommendations were adopted by the committee at the 1928 meeting. These recommendations were concerned primarily with working conditions, such as proper ventilation, along with some shielding recommendations.

Representatives of several countries, including the United States, were invited to attend the Stockholm meeting for the purpose of forming a truly international radiation protection committee. Unfortunately, three major radiologic societies existed in the United States at that time—the American Roentgen Ray Society, the Radium Society, and the Radiological Society of North America—among which there was no unified position in regard to protection criteria. At the suggestion of the ICRP, a single committee was formed. It consisted of members recommended by the three societies and the National Bureau of Standards under the title The Advisory Committee on X-ray and Radium Protection. After World War II, the committee was enlarged and given the name National Committee on Radiation Protection,[7] later changed to the National Council on Radiation Protection and Measurements (NCRP). The first handbook published by the Advisory Committee was noteworthy in that it went into considerably greater detail than did the ICRP recommendations and included such topics as the use of acetate rather than nitrate film (because of fire hazards) and resuscitation techniques for electrical shock caused by high-voltage equipment in use.[8] Three lives are known to have been saved by resuscitation as a direct result of the availability of this handbook.[5]

In 1934, the Advisory Committee put forth the first recommended tolerance dose. It was based on the one-hundredth erythema dose in 30 days, but it took into account the number of actual work hours in a month, with the resulting figure halved as an extra safety factor.[3] This procedure resulted in a recommended tolerance dose of 0.1 R/day. Through similar but not identical reasoning in the same year, the ICRP arrived at a dose of 0.2 R/day.[9]

INTERNAL EMITTERS

By the 1930s there was a recognized need for standards for protection from internal emitters. Although radioactivity was discovered in 1896, it did not catch the public's fancy as immediately as did x-rays. But by the 1930s many tonics containing radium were being sold to the public, and a number of deaths were attributed to these products.[10] The experiences of the radium dial painters and early radium chemists were certainly as tragic as those of the pioneers of x-ray work. In 1941 a National Bureau of Standards Advisory Committee recommended a maximum residual body burden of 0.1 μg of radium.[11] This figure is still used as a radiation protection guide for radium deposited specifically in bone.[4]

MANHATTAN PROJECT

During the period 1942–1945 the crash program (code-named Manhattan Project) to develop the A bomb presented unique radiation protection problems. Large-scale animal experiments were carried out in the national laboratories such as Oak Ridge.[5] Results of these experiments indicated in general that the 0.1-R/day tolerance dose suggested by the Advisory Committee was reasonable. The possible genetic effects of radiation were of some concern, but the danger was considered negligible, since only a small fraction of the population was exposed. The radium burden suggested by the Advisory Committee was used as the basis for the allowable body burden of plutonium.

Health physicists of the Manhattan District made many contributions to modern radiation protection. The concept of the rem, practical monitoring instruments and administrative procedures for large-scale personnel dosimetry, environmental monitoring, and waste disposal were all developed along modern guidelines. One contribution of at least historic significance was the design of the radiation warning symbol as it is used today (Fig. 1). Army Corporal Myron B. Hawkins had drawn the symbol, in its current form, for use on shipments of isotopes from the Oak Ridge Laboratory. Apparently he was aware of similar designs being used at the Berkeley Isotopes Laboratory. In any case, he has been called the Betsy Ross of radiation protection.[3]

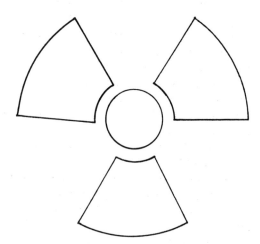

Figure 1. The international radiation warning symbol.

POST-WORLD WAR II PERIOD

During the first postwar meeting of the NCRP, a number of new policy decisions were made.[12] It was decided to lower the permissible dose by a factor of about 2 to 0.3 R/week and to specify the sensitive area of the body to which it applies (i.e., the blood-forming organs). The permissible dose was to be set higher for the skin and higher still for the hands and feet in recognition of lesser sensitivity of these areas. Also, a larger dose was permitted for persons over 45 years of age than for younger workers. Finally, factors were suggested for the relative biologic effectiveness (RBE) of x-rays, γ-rays, β-rays, α-particles, and fast and slow neutrons. The RBE values permitted comparison of the biologic effects of the several types of radiation and were an outgrowth of the war experience with radiation from atomic weapons. Henceforth, because of the RBE factor, all types of ionizing radiation could be characterized in units of rem. The ICRP met in 1950 and echoed the major decisions of the NCRP although not in such great detail.[13]

By 1958, the concept of "tolerance dose" was considered by the NCRP to be unsupportable. In the interval since the last report of the NCRP, an advisory committee, formed by the United Nations and by the National Academy of Sciences,[14] had examined the genetic effects of radiation. It was considered prudent at this time to limit occupational exposure to 5 rem/year and to limit exposure of the general public to 0.5 rem/year.[15] Various provisions were made for the age at which occupational exposure occurs and for slight overexposures in a given year, as long as low cumulative limits were maintained.

To advise the various federal agencies involved in radiation protection standards, the Federal Radiation Council (FRC) was created in 1959.[4] Recommendations of the FRC were released in 1960 and were essentially those of the NCRP. In addition, an extra provision stated that the whole-body dose averaged over the U.S. population should not exceed 0.17 rem/person/year, excluding background and medical radiation. Individuals in the population could still receive 0.5 rem/year.[4] In 1970 the Environmental Protection Agency (EPA) was created and the FRC was dissolved.[16] Although the EPA was given the FRC's policy-setting power, the recommendations made in 1960 have been on the whole unchanged to date.

The history of radiation protection and standards has shown a decrease of recommended exposure limits over the years. There are two reasons for this decrease. First, there has been an increased awareness of the biological effects of radiation. Second, advances in technology have made it possible to use radiation more efficiently while decreasing unnecessary dose to workers and the public. Thus it is now possible to maintain much smaller dose limits than in the early years. Current radiation protection philosophy is based on the assumption that there is no completely "safe" amount of radiation. In practical terms, however, there is certainly a level below which the measurement of biologic effects becomes meaningless. The important operational concept as put forth by the ICRP in 1977[17] is that exposure of an individual should be kept As Low as Reasonably Achievable (the ALARA principle) below recommended limits. In other words, recognizing that there are many situations in which it is impossible to reduce exposure to zero, one must weigh the cost of designing equipment and structures that reduce exposure below the recommended limits against the perceived benefits of doing so. The concept of ALARA will continue to provide a guiding philosophy for professionals in the field of radiation protection as new problems arise.

A chronology of the major events in the history of radiation protection standards and agencies is included at the back of this chapter. It is by no means complete. The interested reader might wish to examine, in particular, two excellent sources (references 3 and 5,) which contain further details and present first-person accounts written by the principals of the era.

REFERENCES

1. Edison TA, Morton W, Tesla N, et al: Effect of x-rays upon the eye. *Nature* 1896; 53:421.
2. Brown P: *American Martyrs to Science Through the Roentgen Rays*. Springfield, III, Charles C Thomas, 1936.
3. Kathren RL, Ziemer PL (eds): *Health Physics: A Backward Glance*. New York, Pergamon Press, 1980.
4. GAO: *Problems in Assessing the Cancer Risks of Low Level Ionizing Radiation Exposure*. Report to the Congress of the United States, vol II. Washington DC, United States General Accounting Office, 1981.
5. Taylor LS: *Radiation Protection Standards*. Cleveland, The Chemical Rubber Company Press, 1971.
6. Report of Second International Congress of Radiology. *Acta Radiol* 1929; Suppl 3: 60.
7. Taylor LS: Brief history of National Committee on Radiation Protection. *Health Phys* 1958; 1:3.
8. NCRP: *X-ray Protection*. NCRP Report 1 (NBS-HB15). Washington DC, 1931.
9. International recommendations for x-ray and radium protection. *Radiology* 1934; 23:682.
10. Evans RD: Radium in man. *Health Phys* 1974; 27:497.
11. NBS: *Safe Handling of Radioactive Luminous Compound*. NBS Handbook 27. Washington DC, National Bureau of Standards, 1941.
12. NCRP: *Medical X-ray Protection Up to Two Million Volts*. NBS Handbook 41. Washington DC, National Bureau of Standards, 1949.
13. ICRP: International recommendations on radiological protection. *Radiology* 1951; 56:432.
14. NAS-NRC: *The Biological Effects of Atomic Radiation*. Summary Reports from a Study by the NAS. Washington DC, National Academy of Sciences-Nuclear Regulatory Commission, 1956.

15. NCRP: Maximum permissible radiation exposures to man. *Radiology* 1958; 71:263.
16. 35, Federal register, 15623 (October 6, 1970).
17. ICRP: *Radiation Protection*. ICRP Publ 26. Oxford, Pergamon, 1977.

CHRONOLOGY OF MAJOR EVENTS IN THE HISTORY OF RADIATION PROTECTION AGENCIES AND STANDARDS

1895	X-rays are discovered by Wilhelm Roentgen.
1896	Various reports of adverse health effects of x-rays begin surfacing. E. Thomson purposely exposes a finger to a large dose of x-rays.
1902	Death of one of Thomas Edison's assistants is related to x-ray exposure.
1913	German Roentgen Ray Society makes the first formal safety recommendations.
1915	British Roentgen Society suggests safety standards.
1920	Deaths from exposure to radium are reported. French Academy of Sciences Study Commission is formed.
1925	Tolerance dose is estimated independently by several researchers; 1/100 erythema dose per month. First International Congress of Radiology is formed. International Commission on Radiation Units and Measurements is formed.
1928	Second International Congress of Radiology officially adopts the roentgen as a unit of radiation. International Committee on X-ray and Radium Protection (ICRP) is formed. Advisory Committee on X-ray and Radium Protection (ACXRP) is formed.
1934	ACXRP recommends tolerance dose of 0.1 R/day. ICRP recommends 0.2 R/day.
1941	National Bureau of Standards Advisory Committee recommends a maximum residual body burden of 0.1 μg radium.
1942–1945	Manhattan Project is started as a crash program to develop the A bomb.
1949	NCRP recommends maximum permissible dose (MPD) of 0.3 R/week.
1950	ICRP recommends maximum permissible dose (MPD) of 0.3 R/week.
1958	NCRP recommends MPD of 5 rem/year occupational and 0.5 rem/year for the general public.
1959	Federal Radiation Council (FRC) is formed; recommends MPD of 0.17 rem/year average exposure for the general public.
1970	FRC is dissolved. Environmental Protection Agency is formed.
1977	ICRP: *A*s *L*ow *A*s *R*easonably *A*chievable (the ALARA principle)

18.

Current Radiation Protection Standards and Concerns

Marc Edwards

A "standard" is that entity established by authority, custom, or general consent as a model or criterion. In the case of radiation protection, one can further discern two broad categories of standards: (1) advisory standards, often put forth as recommendations, which are usually formulated by various commissions, groups, and societies professionally or scientifically concerned with radiation protection; and (2) legal standards, put forth in statutes and regulations, which are formulated by legislative and administrative bodies as well as interpreted and modified by court decisions. As has been pointed out by Taylor,[1] the formulation of radiation protection standards involves both scientific and political processes, each having its own problems and paradigms. This chapter briefly reviews both the advisory and legal standards, attempts to highlight the origin and content of some of the more important concerns, and finally outlines recent attempts at solutions.

Since the history of radiation protection agencies is reviewed in Chapter 17, this chapter discusses only those groups that currently have a large role in the standards-setting process. At the national level, the preeminent advisory organization is the National Council on Radiation Protection and Measurements (NCRP). Formed more than 50 years ago, the NCRP seeks to encourage leading experts and members of the scientific community to analyze and disseminate to the public a wide range of information pertinent to radiation protection. As of 1981, the NCRP had issued 68 reports, many dealing directly with radiation protection standards. The NCRP also collaborates with other organizations, professional societies, and government agencies concerned with radiation protection. An abbreviated list contains such organizations as the American College of Radiology (ACR), American Association of Physicists in Medicine (AAPM), American Nuclear Society (ANS), Atomic Industrial Forum (AIF), Health Physics Society (HPS), Radiological Society of North America (RSNA), Nuclear Regulatory Commission (NRC), and the Environmental Protection Agency (EPA). The

National Academy of Sciences, particularly through sponsorship of the Biological Effects of Ionizing Radiation (BEIR) Committee, has a significant impact on protection standards as well. At the international level, the International Commission on Radiation Protection (ICRP) has produced 33 publications dealing with radiation protection. With the exception of the NRC and EPA, all of these organizations are advisory, although their recommendations are sometimes adopted without much change by legislative and administrative agencies.

Legal standards are set by federal, state, and local government bodies and, through the process of litigation and precedent, by federal and state judicial systems. In a recent article,[1] Taylor listed 17 federal agencies, overseen to one degree or another by 24 congressional committees, that have an impact on federal standards and rules. Prominent among these agencies are the Nuclear Regulatory Commission (NRC), Environmental Protection Agency (EPA), Food and Drug Administration (FDA), Occupational Safety and Health Administration (OSHA), Department of Transportation (DOT), and the General Accounting Office (GAO). States that agree to handle their own radiation safety, rather than be governed by federal law, must establish state laws that are at least as stringent as those at the federal level. Furthermore, any state can establish laws that are more encompassing than federal laws. Several large cities have also attempted further control by local statutes. Finally, the court system can have considerable impact by its power to interpret laws and set precedents. An example of this is the recent ruling by the U.S. Appeals Court that the NRC must consider psychological stress as a form of nuclear power pollution in assessing the environmental impact of nuclear power production.[2]

Examination of the various advisory and legal standards indicates three broad categories: standards for individuals and populations, standards for equipment and facilities, and standards for proper procedure. Under the first category are included individual and group dose limits for the occupationally exposed, the general public, and special subgroups such as the embryo and fetus. The second category includes radiation safety performance standards for individual units of equipment, such as a diagnostic x-ray set, or an entire facility, such as a nuclear reactor. The final category includes standards for proper management, record keeping, monitoring, transportation, and so forth, which, if followed, will help maintain safety. Legal implementation of radiation safety standards is often achieved through the mechanism of licensure, either to individuals or to institutions. Failure to meet safety standards can result in a loss of the license or in economic penalties. Unlike legal standards, recommended standards are promulgated through continuing education of personnel concerned with radiation safety, and implementation is largely dependent on voluntary action.

The task of reviewing current standards is far too lengthy for this discussion. Even a simple cataloging of significant standards would take hundreds of pages. Instead, a single example is given to illustrate the significant issues. Suited to this purpose is the radiation protection standard for maximum permissible dose (MPD) equivalent to an occupationally exposed person, a member of the general public and the population as a whole. This subject was reviewed by the NCRP in 1971 and 1975[3,4] and by the ICRP in 1977.[5] The recommendations of these groups, together with selected federal rules and proposals influenced by them, are shown in Table 1. The most significant change from the earlier NCRP Report 39 limits to the later ICRP Report 26 limits is the abandonment of the MPD and maximum permissible concentration (MPC) system in favor of "dose-equivalent limits." The MPD–MPC methodology grew out of the concept that "critical organs" determine the radiation detriment. The critical organ was defined as that part of the body most susceptible to radiation damage under the specific conditions considered. With the realization that any organ can contribute to potential risk, the more recent ICRP report 26 recommendations use the "summed weighted-sites from all sources" method. Although the 5-rem limit remains unchanged, contributions from both external and internal doses to all organs, not just a few "critical organs," are explicitly considered. The whole-body external dose equivalent is obtained by multiplying each organ dose by a given weighting factor and summing over all organs. The internal dose equivalent is calculated using annual limit on intake (ALI) activities, as discussed in ICRP Report 30.[6] Hence the 5-rem/year limit is met if

$$\frac{\sum\limits_{i} W_i H_i}{5} + \sum\limits_{j} \frac{I_j}{(ALI)_j} \leqslant 1 \tag{1}$$

where W_i is the weighting factor for organ i, H_i is the external dose equivalent to organ i, 5 is the annual limit in rems, I_j is the annual intake of isotope j, and $(ALI)_j$ is the annual limit on intake of isotope j.

Individual organ weighting factors can be used to infer possible organ MPDs if no other organ is irradiated. For instance, since the weighting factor for the breast is 0.15, the maximum permissible breast dose is $5/0.15 = 33$ rem. However, if the breast was exposed to this level, no additional exposure to the breast or to any other organ should be allowed, since this would exceed the recommendations described in Equation (1). In no case is a single organ permitted to exceed a nonstochastic effect dose limit of 50 rem.

Another significant departure from NCRP recommendations is the abandonment of genetic and somatic population dose limits. These dose limits were considered unnecessary, as there has been no indication that the 0.17-rem/year population limits are likely to be exceeded if the 5-rem/year

TABLE 1. SUMMARY OF RADIATION PROTECTION GUIDELINES AND STANDARDS AS IMPLEMENTED BY VARIOUS ORGANIZATIONS

	NCRP
MAXIMUM PERMISSIBLE DOSE EQUIVALENT FOR OCCUPATIONAL EXPOSURE	
Combined whole body occupational exposure	
Prospective annual limit	5 rems in any 1 yr.
Retrospective annual limit	10–15 rems in any 1 yr.
Long term accumulation	(N–18) x 5, where N is age in years
Skin	15 rems in any 1 yr.
Hands	75 rems in any 1 yr. (25/qtr.)
Forearms	30 rems in any 1 yr. (10/qtr.)
Other organs, tissues and organ systems	15 rems in 1 yr. (5/qtr.)
	Gonads
	Red bone marrow } 5 rems in
	Lens of eye } any 1 yr.
Fertile women	0.5 rem in gestation period
DOSE LIMITS FOR PUBLIC, OR OCCASIONALLY EXPOSED INDIVIDUALS	
Individual or Occasional	0.5 rem in any 1 yr.
POPULATION DOSE LIMITS	
Genetic	0.17 rem average per yr.
Somatic	0.17 rem average per yr.

[a] ICRP Report 26 guidelines specifically involve both externally and internally deposited dose in the 5-rem/year guideline.
[b] Dose limits given here are derived from the relative organ weighting factors assuming all dose is deposited in the particular organ and nowhere else.
[c] Dose limit identical to that in ICRP Report 26.
[d] Dose limits inferred from organ weighting factors.

occupational and 0.5-rem/year general public limits are followed. For similar reasons, quarterly and lifetime dose equivalent limits were also abandoned.

The response of the federal regulatory agencies to recommendations of the NCRP and ICRP has been varied. Numerical recommendations, such as whole-body and organ dose limits, have often been closely followed. As seen

ICRP 26	Current 10 CFR 20	Proposed EPA Radiation Protection Guidance
5 rems in a yr. from all sources[a]	5 rems in any 1 yr	5 rems in a yr. from all sources[c]
Same as prospective	12 rems in any 1 yr.	Same as prospective
None other than implied by prospective annual limit	(N-18) x 5 rems, where N is age in years	100 rem lifetime
50 rems in a yr.	30 rems in any 1 yr.	
50 rems in a yr.	75 rems in any 1	50 rems in a yr.
50 rems in a yr.	75 rems in any 1 yr.	30 rems in a yr.
Gonads[b] 20 rems/any 1 yr. Breast 33 rems/any 1 yr. Red bone marrow 42 rems/any 1 yr. Lung 42 rems/any 1 yr. Lens of eye 30 rems/any 1 yr.	Gonads Red bone marrow } 5 rems in any 1 yr. Lens of eye	Gonads 5 rems/yr. Breast[a] 25 rems/yr. Red bone marrow[d] 30 rems/yr. Thyroid 30 rems/yr. Lung 30 rems/yr. Lens of eyes 5 rems/yr.
0.5 rem in gestation period	0.5 rem in gestation period recommended	0.5 rem in gestation period
0.5 rem in a yr.	0.5 rem in a yr.	Not addressed
Not considered necessary	Not addressed	Not addressed
Not considered necessary	Not addressed	Not addressed

in Table 1, the current version of NRC regulations for radiation protection published in the Code of Federal Regulations[7] is very similar to limits set forth in the NCRP Report 39. A major revision of this section of the code (10 CFR 20), which is currently undergoing development,[8] adopts the ICRP Report 26 recommendations, as well as the ICRP Report 30 concepts of dose limits, as briefly discussed above. A recent proposal by the EPA to establish new radiation protection guidelines for federal agencies[9] appears to follow ICRP methodology roughly, with the exception that it adopts the lower of individual organ dose limitations proposed by the NCRP or ICRP (Table 1).

Divergence between recommendation and regulation more often occurs in the area of "good practice" or "proper procedure." Nowhere is this more apparent than in the controversy over ALARA. Since their inception, all radiation protection recommendations have urged that, regardless of numerical limits, it is always desirable to keep exposures As Low As Reasonably Practicable (ALAP), or As Low As Reasonably Achievable (ALARA). This viewpoint was further reinforced by adoption of the linear no-threshold risk-estimation model, in which there is no "safe" amount of radiation. Viewed as a call to exercise judicious restraint in dealing with radiation, the principle of ALARA is not the least bit controversial. To a regulatory agency, however, a philosophic principle is often viewed as an unenforceable "wish" in dire need of codification. A review of occupational exposure records also indicated that only a small fraction of workers actually receive an annual dose close to the recommended limit, with the average dose in many cases being approximately 1 rem/year. To a large degree, ALARA was being achieved. Since one way of assuring success is to mandate it, the concept of "that which is achievable is required" arose in the form of regulated "action levels" or "reference levels." Such levels, although specifically stated not to be limits, are those dose levels that, if exceeded or anticipated to be exceeded, require some sort of response to be initiated. The proposed values of reference levels range from one-twentieth to one-fifth the values of annual dose limits. Concern has been expressed that such a codified system guaranteeing ALARA may result in de facto lower annual dose limits and higher radiation protection costs, but with little actual improvement over current radiation protection performance.

One possible approach to deciding when "sufficient" protection has been achieved is to require a rigorous cost/benefit analysis of specific dose levels in specific situations.[5] While this approach is attractive in principle, it is beset with practical problems.[10] It assumes that the risks of radiation exposure can be quantified accurately, that the benefits of radiation exposure can be quantified accurately, and that both can be expressed in an equivalent, usually monetary, value system. It also implicitly assumes, or hopes, that an equally rational methodology is used to assess nonradiogenic risks such that no undue burden is placed on radiation risk control as opposed to all others. All these assumptions are currently unfulfilled, such that cost/benefit analysis as a mechanism of regulatory dose limitation is unlikely to gain acceptance in the near future.

One potential solution to the regulatory problems presented by adopting the "no-threshold, hence no-safe-limit" philosophy is the establishment of "de minimis" levels.[11] The terminology, derived from the maxim *de minimis non curat lex* (i.e., "the law does not concern itself with trifles"), indicates a "practical threshold" beneath which any consequence is decided to be of no importance. This viewpoint recognizes the fact that, while there may be no absolutely safe amount of radiation, surely a point is reached at which the potential detriment is comparatively minuscule and therefore can and should be ignored. The problem then becomes by what criteria and at what level should the de minimis level be set. If set too low, it would do little to alleviate regulatory problems; if set too high, it might result in poor radiation safety practice. Perhaps as an example of the former case, the current proposal for the completely revised NRC standards (10 CFR 20) suggests a de minimis level of 0.1 mrem/year.[8] Other proposals[11] suggest a reasonable fraction of normal background radiation or a level at which the projected risk is equivalent to other normal nonradiogenic risks.

The final radiation protection "concern" discussed in this chapter is that of medical radiation exposure. It is often not realized, even by members of the medical community, that there is no regulatory limit to the amount of radiation that a patient can receive in the course of a medical procedure. Regulated occupational or nonoccupational radiation exposure accounts for less than 1 percent of the average yearly U.S. population exposure; in contrast, medical exposure accounts for approximately 50 percent, and background radiation accounts for the remainder. Even assuming that all medical exposure is justifiable from medical and risk/benefit considerations, it is desirable that medical procedures be performed with as low an exposure as necessary. Although this has long been a tenet of good practice for radiologists, studies have shown that the average exposure for identical examinations at different institutions has a very wide variance and that a significant fraction of studies may be performed for other than medical reasons.

Since they clearly could not dictate dose limits for individual patients, the regulatory agencies, particularly the Bureau of Radiological Health,* chose instead to regulate equipment performance with the intent of increasing dose efficiency. Title 21, Part 1000 of the Code of Federal Regulations[12] established requirements for such items as beam limitation, filtration, leakage, and maximum exposure rates for new equipment. The Bureau of Radiological Health has also become very active in promoting quality assurance and public awareness programs of risk/benefit considerations in radiologic procedures. A recent program seeks to define and promulgate referral criteria for diagnostic procedures that have a potential for misapplication. More controversial regulations, often occurring at the state level, involve setting dose limits for typical examinations and requiring state licensure of allied health professionals. Ultimately, the responsibility of effective dose utilization in diagnostic radiology must continue to reside with the professionals involved in that specialty. However, every effort should be made to

---

*Recently the name of this agency was changed to the National Center for Diseases and Radiological Health.

ensure that they are educationally and ethically prepared to make decisions in the best interests of the patient.

REFERENCES

1. Taylor LS: Some nonscientific influences on radiation protection standards and practices. *Health Phys* 1980; 39:851–874.
2. NRC must weigh psychic costs. *Science* 1982; 216: 1203–1204.
3. NCRP: *Basic Radiation Protection Criteria.* NCRP Report 39. Washington DC, National Council on Radiation Protection and Measurements, 1971.
4. *Review of the Current State of Radiation Protection Philosophy.* NCRP Report 43. Washington DC, NCRP: National Council on Radiation Protection and Measurement. 1975.
5. ICRP: *Recommendations of the ICRP.* ICRP Publ 26. International Commission on Radiation Protection. New York, Pergamon, 1977.
6. ICRP: *Limits for Intakes of Radionuclides by Workers.* ICRP Publ 30. International Commission on Radiation Protection. New York, Pergamon, 1979.
7. Standards for protection against radiation (10 CFR 20). *Federal Register* 1981.
8. Working document of proposed revision (10 CFR 20). *Federal Register.* Private communication with NRC.
9. EPA: Federal radiation protection guidance for occupational exposures; proposed recommendations. *Federal Register.* 1981; 46: Vol. no. 15, 7836–7844.
10. ICRP: *Implications of Commission Recommendations that Doses be Kept as Low as Readily Achievable.* ICRP Publ 22. International Commission on Radiation Protection. New York, Pergamon, 1974.
11. Eisenbud M: The Concept of de minimis dose. In *Quantitative Risk in Standards Setting.* Proceedings of the 16th Annual Meeting of NCRP, NCRP Proc No 2. Washington DC, 1980.
12. Performance standards for ionizing radiation emitting products (21 CFR 1000). *Federal Register* 1981.

19.

Modification of Radiation Damage by Naturally Occurring Substances

Kedar N. Prasad

The major objectives of studying the modification of radiation sensitivity have been (1) to identify a compound that will produce a differential protection or sensitization of the effect of irradiation on normal and tumor tissue, and (2) to understand more about the mechanisms of radiation damage.

In spite of massive research on this particular problem since World War II, the first objective remains elusive. During this period, numerous radio-protective and radiosensitizing agents have been identified.[1-3] These agents have served as important biologic tools for increasing our understanding of radiation injuries. Most of these substances are synthetic compounds and are very toxic to humans. In addition, very few of the compounds provide differential modifications of the effect of radiation on tumor and normal cells. This chapter presents objectives for identifying naturally occurring substances that modify the effect of x-irradiation on mammalian cells and discusses the role of physiologic substances in modifying radiation injuries on mammalian normal and tumor cells.

CYCLIC NUCLEOTIDES

Cyclic nucleotides, adenosine 3′,5′-cyclic monophosphate (cAMP), and guanosine 3′,5′-cyclic monophosphate (cGMP) occur in all mammalian cells and are formed by catalyzing adenosine triphosphate (ATP) and guanosine triphosphate (GTP) with adenylate cyclase and guanylate cyclase, respectively. cAMP and cGMP are degraded by cAMP phosphodiesterase and cGMP phosphodiesterase, respectively. Numerous studies[4-6] have shown that cyclic nucleotides are involved in the regulation of growth, differentiation, and malignancy of certain cell types. Since the rate of proliferation and the degree of differentiation are important factors in determining the radio-sensitivity of mammalian cells, the obvious question is whether cyclic nucleo-tides would modify the radiation response of normal cells and tumor cells.

In 1972, it was reported[7] for the first time that prostaglandin E_1 (PGE_1), a stimulator of adenylate cyclase, and 4- (3-butoxy-4-methoxybenzyl)-2-imidazolidine (R020-1724), an inhibitor of cyclic nucleotide phosphodi-esterase, increased the survival of x-irradiated Chinese hamster ovary (CHO-K_1) cells by about two-fold, provided they were given before irradiation. Both PGE_1 and R020-1724 were ineffective when given after irradiation. On the basis of this study, it was postulated that the level of inter-cellular cAMP might be inversely related to the radiosensitivity of mam-malian cells.[7] Although the level of intracellular cAMP was not measured in the initial study,[7] other investigators have shown that the level of cAMP in CHO-K_1 cells increases after treatment with PGE_1 and inhibitors of cyclic nucleotide phosphodiesterase.[8] The basic observation on the radioprotective role of cAMP has been confirmed and extended by several investigators. For example, it has been shown that cAMP-stimulating agents, when given before x-irradiation, increase the survival of irradiated Chinese hamster V-79 [9,10] and thymocyte[11] cells in culture. It has also been reported that cAMP-stimulating agents reduce x-ray-induced mitotic delay in human kidney T cells[12] and in S-180 ascites tumor cells.[13] Most of these studies did not deter-mine the level of cAMP in the cells before irradiation. It has been further suggested[9] that changes in cAMP during the cell cycle could be one of the important factors responsible for the variation in radiosensitivity as a function of stages of the cell cycle. One study[10] has reported that cells with an increased level of cAMP become more sensitive to irradiation at higher radiation doses, but exhibit increased resistance at lower doses. The precise reason for this observation is unknown.

Other investigators[14] have reported that adenosine triphosphate (ATP), 5-adenosine monophosphate (5'-AMP), and 3'-adenosine monophosphate (3-AMP), when given singly before irradiation, provide a significant degree of protection in irradiated mice. cAMP by itself is ineffective, but in com-bination with ATP it provides a higher degree of protection (70 percent) than that obtained with ATP alone (44 percent). The combination of 3'-AMP with 5'-AMP produces 100 percent survival.[14] On the basis of these data, it has been suggested that a number of radioprotective agents might mediate their effects via cAMP. However, exogenous cAMP generally does not pene-trate the cell membrane. In addition, it is rapidly hydrolyzed to 5'-AMP in plasma. Similarly, exogenous ATP does not generally enter the cell mem-brane, so that the radioprotective effect of the above agents might be mediated by an indirect effect of the compounds, and not by cAMP.

Two recent studies have confirmed the involvement of cAMP in the mechanisms of radiation protection in vivo; dibutyryl cAMP protects hair follicles[15] and gut stem cells [15,16] against radiation-induced cell death, without protecting lymphosarcoma and breast carcinoma.[15] This is an intriguing observation, because it is one of the few examples in which a physiologic substance protects normal tissue without protecting tumor tissue. If similar results are observed in human tissue, an elevation of the intracellular level of cAMP during radiation therapy might improve the effectiveness of the therapy by protecting the normal tissue. It is well known that the damage of normal tissue is the limiting factor in radiation therapy of tumors.

IS cAMP INVOLVED IN MEDIATING THE RADIOPROTECTIVE EFFECTS OF DIVERSE AGENTS?

It is well known that hypoxic cells are very resistant to x-irradiation. It has recently been reported[17] that the intracellular level of cAMP markedly increases in moderately hypoxic cells and therefore the radioresistance of hypoxic cells could be related in part to a rise in cellular cAMP. It also appears that the radioprotective effect of sulfhydryl compounds might be mediated in part by cAMP. For example, cysteamine, a well-known radioprotective agent, increases the intracellular level of cAMP in the liver 15 minutes after administration.[18] The level of cAMP in proliferating tissue after administration of cysteamine has not been measured. Therefore, one cannot be certain as to whether the rise in the cAMP level of proliferating tissue is associated with radiation protection. Since cysteamine is known to produce hypoxia, a rise is expected in the intracellular level of cAMP after treatment with cysteamine. Preincubation of mouse bone marrow cells with PGE_1 (a stimulator of adenylate cyclase), cAMP, and cGMP before the addition of cysteamine increases the radioprotective effect of cysteamine.[19] Unfortunately, the intracellular level of cAMP has not been measured under the above experimental conditions. In addition, the rationale for the addition of cAMP and cGMP in these studies has not been provided.

Although some in vitro and in vivo data suggest that the level of cAMP could be one of the important factors in the radiosensitivity of mammalian cells, the role of cGMP on the radiosensitivity of mammalian cells remains completely unknown. The availability of analogues of cGMP and stimulators of guanylate cyclase makes it possible to investigate this problem. Further in vitro and in vivo studies are indicated on the role of cAMP and cGMP in the radiosensitivity of normal and tumor cells.

BUTYRIC ACID

Butyric acid, a 4-carbon fatty acid, occurs naturally in the body and is formed by the hydrolysis of ethyl butyrate. Recent studies show that these fatty acids affect morphology, growth rate, and gene expression in several

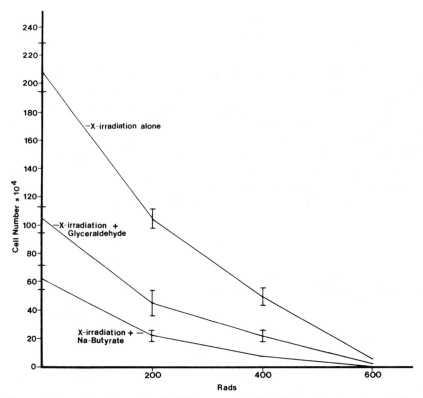

Figure 1. Neuroblastoma cells (50,000) were plated in Falcon plastic culture dishes (60 mm). Sodium butyrate (0.5 m*M*) and DL-glyceraldehyde (0.25 m*M*) were added immediately after various doses of x-irradiation. Each value represents an average of at least six samples. The bar at each point is the standard elevation. The vertical bars of the points not shown in figure were too small to be indicated. (From Prasad KN: Control mechanisms of malignancy and differentiation in cultures of nerve cells. In Evans AE (ed): *Advances in Neuroblastoma Research.* New York, Raven Press, 1980, pp 135–144.)

mammalian tumor cells in culture.[20-21] In addition, sodium butyrate enhances the growth inhibitory effect of x-irradiation on mouse neuroblastoma cells in culture (Fig. 1). Sodium butyrate inhibits anaerobic glycolysis by reducing lactic acid dehydrogenase activity.[22] Since neuroblastoma cells are more sensitive to inhibitors of anaerobic glycolysis than are other cell types,[23] sodium butyrate-induced cell death and enhancement of radiation response might be partly related to the inhibition of anaerobic glycolysis. Supporting this observation is the finding that DL-glyceraldehyde, an inhibitor of anaerobic glycolysis, also inhibits the growth and increases the radiation response of neuroblastoma cells in culture (Fig. 1).

Sodium butyrate is nontoxic in humans. Doses of 7-10 g/day produce no clinically detectable toxic effect in patients with neuroblastomas (T. Voute and L. Furman, personal communication, 1979). Further in vitro and in vivo studies should be performed to evaluate the role of inhibitors of anaerobic glycolysis in modifying radiation response.

VITAMINS

Vitamin C

In vitro data suggest that vitamin C (sodium ascorbate) modifies the effects of x-irradiation on the survival of mammalian cells in culture. The extent of modification depends on the type of cell. For example, sodium ascorbate increases the growth inhibitory effects of x-irradiation on mouse neuroblastoma cells in culture,[24] whereas it protects Chinese hamster ovary cells.[25] Vitamin C does not modify the effect of x-irradiation on rat glioma (C-6) cells in culture.[24] A preliminary study[26] has shown that vitamin C, when combined with ionizing radiation, increases the survival of mice with ascites tumor cells in comparison with those treated with x-irradiation alone. Dehydroascorbate, a metabolite of vitamin C, produces cytotoxic effects primarily on hypoxic Chinese hamster lung cells in culture and enhances the effect of ionizing radiation on Ehrlich ascites cells in vivo.[27] Since the hypoxic cells are known to be highly radioresistant, the addition of vitamin C during radiation therapy may be more effective in killing hypoxic cells by dehydroascorbate. The effectiveness of this mechanism depends on the proportion of hypoxic cells in the tumor mass at the time of vitamin C treatment. More experimental work is needed to evaluate the role of sodium ascorbate and dehydroascorbate in modifying the radiation response of normal and tumor cells.

Vitamin A

Pretreatment of animals with vitamin A (retinol) increases the growth inhibitory effect of x-irradiation on mammary adenocarcinoma, L1210 leukemia, and a fibrosarcoma.[28-31] The administration of vitamin A alone does not affect the growth of these tumors. Retinol also causes inhibition of DNA repair processes in ultraviolet (UV)-irradiated lymphocytes.[32] This finding suggests that vitamin A-induced enhancement of the effect of x-irradiation on tumor cells might be caused by the inhibitory effect of retinol on DNA repair processes.[32] More studies are needed to evaluate the role of retinal and analogues of retinoic acid in modifying the radiation response of normal and tumor cells.

Vitamin E

Studies on the radioprotective effect of vitamin E have produced conflicting results,[33-45] probably because of differences in doses and types of vitamin E, doses of radiation, administration route, and administration time. Experimental results of various studies are listed in Tables 1 and 2. Very few of

TABLE 1. Modification of Effects of Ionizing Radiation by α-Tocopherol and Its Esters in Whole Animals

Animals	Type	Dose (mg/kg)	Route	Injection Schedules	Radiation dose (rad)	Observations
Mice	α-T ac[a]	15	Oral	0.036% diet −1 wk + 30 days	650, 750, 850	Increase in survival[33]
Rats	α-T[b]	60	Oral	−2 to +1 day	700	No effect on survival[34]
Mice	α-T	300	IM[d]	−5 to +5 day	700	Marginal increase in survival[35]
Male mice	α-T aq[c]	25−150	IM	0 and until death	550	Ineffective at lower concns. increases mortality at higher concns.[36]
Male mice	Mixed	0.25% diet	Diet	−6 wk to +4 mo	1600 (200/wk)	No effect in life-span[37]
Male mice	α-T or α-T ac	40−600	IP[e]	0 days	500−750	Increase in survival at lower concn.; no effect at higher concn.[38]
Female mice	α-T aq	1000	IP	0 days	400−800	Increased survival at 500, 600, rad[39]
Female mice	α-T	0.01% diet	Diet	Various periods pre- and postirradiation	800	No effect on survival[40]
Female mice	α-T aq	50	IP	Immediate postirradiation (on deficient or normal diet)	800	Increase in survival[40]
Rats	α-T and α-T aq	2.5% diet 600	Diet IP	−2 wk until irradiation and α-T aq 4 h before irradiation	1500−2000 Thoracic	No effect on survival[41]
Male mice	α-T	27,55,82	IP	−1 day	550,650	Increase in survival at lower concn.; no effect at higher concn.[42]

a α-Tocopherol acetate.
b α-Tocopherol.
c α-Tocopherol aqueous preparation.
d Intramuscular.
e Intraperitoneal.
f 0 days, 10–30 minutes before irradiation; (−), before irradiation; (+), after irradiation.

TABLE 2. Modification of Effects of Ionizing Radiation by α-Tocopherol and Esters on Tumor Cells

Animals	Type	Dose (mg/kg)	Route	Injection Schedules (days)	[c]Radiation dose (rad)	Observations
Mice with squamous cells	α-T aq[a]	1000	IP[c]	0	1000–2000 whole body	Increased survival of tumor cells in α-T-treated[39]
Rats with IM tumors	α-T aq	50	IM[d]	−7 or −1	3000 to tumor	Radiation sensitizing effect of α-T ac on tumors[43]
Rats with IM tumors	α-T ac[b] or D-α-T ac	50–1000 37	IM Oral	−7	3000 to tumor	Sensitizing effect due to radiation up to 500 mg, but not with 1000 mg[44]
Mouse neuroblastoma cells in culture	α-T aq	5 μg/ml		3	400	Enhances inhibitory effect[45]

[a]α-Tocopherol aqueous preparation.
[b]α-Tocopherol acetate.
[c]Intraperitoneal
[d]Intramuscular.
[e]0 days, 10–30 min before irradiation; (−), before irradiation, (+), after irradiation.

the studies have measured the cellular level of vitamin E before or after irradiation. There are different forms of vitamin E such as DL-α-tocopherol acetate, DL-α-tocopherol nicotinate, DL-α-tocopherol succinate, D-α-tocopherol acid succinate and DL-α-tocopherol free alcohol. The stability, solubility and cellular uptake of the different forms vary. Therefore, the radioprotective effect of various doses of each form of vitamin E should be identified. The plasma and tissue levels of vitamin E must be determined in separate experiments before irradiation in order to establish the role of vitamin E in modifying the radiation response of mammalian cells.

In vitro studies suggest that the presence of α-tocopherol during irradiation reduces the radiosensitivity of the erythrocyte membrane[46-48]; vitamin E when given after irradiation has no effect. Dietary vitamin E treatment has significantly reversed radiation-induced immunosuppression as measured by the delayed type hypersensitivity response to oxazolene.[33] Vitamin E also reduces the radiation-induced decrease in the activity of cytosol glutathione peroxidase.[33] These studies suggest that the presence of vitamin E modifies the response to radiation at several levels. A systematic study on the role of vitamin E in modifying radiation response is needed before any firm conclusions can be drawn.

CONCLUSIONS

Several physiologic substances (e.g., adenosine, 3',5'-cyclic monophosphate, butyric acid, and vitamins A, C, and E) are known to modify the radiation response of mammalian cells. Most of the studies of these substances have been performed in vitro, leaving their relevance to whole organisms to be ascertained. In addition, it is unknown as to whether all the modifiers selectively modify the radiation response of tumor cells as compared with normal cells. Since all the compounds are relatively nontoxic in humans, they might be important in improving the effectiveness of the radiation therapy of tumors. Extensive experimental work is needed before clinical trials of cAMP, butyric acid, and vitamins in combination with radiation therapy can be considered.

REFERENCES

1. Thomson JF: *Radiation Protection in Mammals.* New York, Reinhold, 1962.
2. Bacq ZM, Alexander P: *Fundamentals of Radiobiology.* New York, Pergamon, 1961.
3. Brady LW (ed): *Radiation Sensitizers: Their Use in Clinical Management of Cancer.* New York, Masson Publishing USA, 1980.

4. Prasad KN: Differentiation of neuroblastoma cells in culture. *Biol Rev* 1975; 50:129–165.

5. Pastan IH, Johnson GS, Anderson WB: Role of cyclic nucleotides in growth control. *Annu Rev Biochem* 1975; 44:491–522.

6. Goldberg ND, Haddox MK, Dunham E, et al: The yig yang hypothesis of biological control: Opposing influences of cyclic GMP and cyclic AMP in the regulation of cell proliferation and other biological processes. In Clarkson B, Baserga R (eds): *Control of Proliferation in Animal Cells.* Cold Spring Harbor, NY, Cold Spring Harbor Laboratory, 1974; pp 609–625.

7. Prasad KN: Radioprotective effect of prostaglandins and an inhibitor of cyclic nucleotide phosphodiesterase in mammalian cells in culture. *Int J Radiat Biol* 1972; 22:187–189.

8. Puck TT: Cyclic AMP, the microtubule–microfilament system, and cancer. *Proc Natl Acad Sci USA* 1977; 74:4491–4495.

9. Lehnert S: Intracellular cyclic AMP levels and radiosensitivity in synchronized V-79 cells. *Radiat Res* 1975; 64:394–398.

10. Lehnert S: Modification of post-irradiation survival of mammalian cells by intracellular cyclic AMP. *Radiat Res* 1975; 62:107–116.

11. Ojeda F, Aravena G, Folch H: Modification of radiation response by agents that elevate the intracellular cAMP level. *Experientia* 1980; 36:857–958.

12. Boynton AL, Evans TC: Investigation of effects of cyclic AMP and related drugs on recovery of radiation induced mitotic delay in mouse ascites tumor cells. *Radiat Res* 1973; 55:595–596.

13. Scaife JF: Cyclic 3′-5′-adenosine monophosphate: Its possible role in mammalian cell mitosis and radiation-induced mitotic G_2 delay. *Int J Radiat Biol* 1971; 19:191–195.

14. Langendorff H, Langendorff M: Chemical radiation protection and the cAMP mechanism. *Int J Radiat Biol* 1971; 19:493–495.

15. Dubravsky NB, Hunter N, Mason K, et al: Dibutyryl cyclic adenosine monophosphate: Effect on radiosensitivity of tumors and normal tissue in mice. *Radiology* 1978; 126:799–802.

16. Lehnert S: Radioprotection of mouse intestine by inhibitors of cyclic AMP phosphodiesterase. *Int J Radiat Oncol Biol Biophys* 1979; 5:825–833.

17. Jacobson EA, Koch CJ, Inch WR, et al: Radiation induced 3′-5′ adenosine monophosphate (cAMP) changes in aerobic and hypoxic mammalian cells. *Proc Am Assoc Cancer Res* 1980; 21:30a.

18. Mitznegg P: On the mechanism of radioprotection by cysteamine II. The significance of cyclic 3′-5′-AMP for the cysteamine induced radioprotection effects in white mice. *Int J Radiat Biol* 1973; 24:339–344.

19. Pazdernik TL, Uyeki EM: Enhancement of the radioprotective effects of 2-mercaptoethylamine on colony forming cells by agents which alter cyclic nucleotide levels. *Int J Radiat Biol* 1974; 26:331–340.

20. Prasad KN: Butyric acid: A small fatty acid with diverse biological functions. *Life Sci* 1980; 27:1351–1358.

21. Prasad KN, Sinha PK: Effect of sodium butyrate on mammalian cells in culture. A review. *In Vitro* 1976; 12:125–131.

22. Prasad KN: Control mechanisms of malignancy and differentiation in cultures of nerve cells. In Evans AE (ed): *Advances in Neuroblastoma Research*. New York, Raven Press, 1980; pp 135-144.

23. Sakamoto A, Prasad KN: Effect of DL-glyceraldehyde on mouse neuroblastoma cell culture. *Cancer Res* 1972; 32:532-534.

24. Prasad KN, Sinha PK, Ramanujam M, et al: Sodium ascorbate potentiates the growth inhibitory effect of certain agents on neuroblastoma cells in culture. *Proc Natl Acad Sci USA* 1979; 76:829-832.

25. O'Connor MK, Malone JF, Moriarty M, et al: A radioprotective effect of vitamin C observed in Chinese hamster ovary cells. *Brit J Radio* 1977; 50:587-591.

26. Tewfik FA, Riley EF, Mital CR: The influence of ascorbic acid on the growth of solid tumors in mice and on tumor control by x-irradiation. Presented at the Annual Meeting of the Radiation Research Society, May 8-12, 1977.

27. Koch CJ, Biaglow JE: Toxicity of radiation sensitivity modification, and metabolic effects of dehydroascorbate and ascorbate in mammalian cells. *J Cell Physiol* 1978; 94:299-306.

28. Tannock IF, Suit DH, Marshal N: Vitamin A and the radiation response of experimental tumors: An immune mediated effect. *J Natl Cancer Inst* 1972; 48:731-741.

29. Cohen MH, Carbone PP: Enhancment of the antitumors effect of 1,3-Bis (2-Chlorethyl) -1-nitrosourea and cyclophosphamide by Vitamin A. *J Natl Cancer Inst* 1972; 48:921-926.

30. Brandes D, Anton E, Lamm KW. Studies of L1210 leukemia. Ultrastructure and cytochemical changes after treatment with cyclophosphamide and vitamin A. *J Natl Cancer Inst* 1967; 39:385-421.

31. Brandes D, Anton E. The role of lysosomes in cellular lytic processes. III. Electron histochemical changes in mammary tumors after treatment with cytoxan and vitamin A. *Lab Invest* 1966; 15:987-1006.

32. Gaudin D, Gregg RS, Yielding KL: DNA repair inhibition: A possible mechanism of action of Co-carcinogens. *Biochem Biophys Res Commun* 1971; 45:630-636.

33. Srinivansan V, Jacobs AK, Simpson SA, et al: Radioprotection by vitamin E: Effect on hepatic enzymes, delayed type hypersensitivity and post-irradiation survival of mice. In Meyskens FL Jr, Prasad KN (eds): *First International Conference on the Modulation and Mediation of Cancer by Vitamins*. Base, S. Karger, 1983.

34. Furth FW, Coulter MP, Howland JW: Failure of alpha tocopherol to protect against radiation injury in the rat. University of Rochester Atomic Energy Report UR-152, 1951; pp 34-38 .

35. Bacq ZM, Herve A: Protection of mice against a lethal dose of x-rays by cyanide, azide and malononitrile. *Br J Radiol* 1951; 24:717-721.

36. Haley TK, McCulloh EF, McCormick WG: Influence of water-soluble vitamin E on survival time in irradiated mice. *Science* 1954; 119:126-127.

37. Ershoff BH, Steers CW Jr: Antioxidants and survival time of mice exposed to multiple sublethal doses of x-irradiation. *Proc Soc Exp Biol Med* 1960; 104:274-276.

38. Huber R, Schöder E: Antioxdantien and Uberlebenstrate ganzkorperbestrahlter Mause. *Strahlentherapie* 1962; 119:308-315.

39. Sakamoto K, Sakka M: Reduced effect of irradiation on normal and malignant cells irradiated in vivo in mice pretreated with vitamin E. *Br J Radiol* 1973; 46:538-540.

40. Malick MA, Roy RM, Sternberg J: Effect of vitamin E on post-irradiation death in mice. *Experientia* 1978; 34:1216-1217.

41. Rostock RA, Stryker JA, Abt AB: Evaluation of high-dose vitamin E as a radioprotective agent. *Radiology* 1980; 136:763-766.

42. Londer HM, Myers CE: Radioprotective effect of vitamin E. *Am J Clin Nutr* 1978; 31:705.

43. Kagerud A, Holm G, Larson H, et al: Tocopherol and local x-ray irradiation of two transplantable rat tumors. *Cancer Lett* 1978; 5:123-129.

44. Kagerud A, Peterson HI: Tocopherol in irradiation of experimental neoplasms. Influence of dose and administration. *Acta Radiol Oncol* 1981; 20:97-100.

45. Prasad KN, Edwards-Prasad J, Ramanujam S, et al: Vitamin E increases the growth inhibitory and differentiating effects of tumor therapeutic agents in neuroblastoma and glioma cells in culture. *Proc Soc Exp Biol Med* 1980; 164:158-163.

46. Prince EW, Little JB: The effect of dietary fatty acids and tocopherol on the radiosensitivity of mammalian erythrocytes. *Radiat Res* 1973; 53:49-64.

47. Hoffer A, Roy RM: Vitamin E decreases erythrocyte fragility after whole-body irradiation. *Radiat Res* 1975; 61:439-443.

48. Konings AWT, Drijver EB: Radiation effect on neuroblastoma. Vitamin E deficiency and lipid peroxidation. *Radiat Res* 1979; 80:494-501.

20.

Legal Recourse for Damages Suffered from Low-Level Radiation Exposure

Marilyn M. Pesto-Edwards

In the past few years several events involving toxic substances have received widespread coverage by the media, thereby alerting an already aware population to the hazards of exposure to toxic agents. Incidents such as Three Mile Island, Love Canal, and Hemlock, Michigan, the exposure plight of veterans to radiation at the Nevada Test Site and to Agent Orange in Vietnam, and the exposure of factory workers to asbestos, have been highly publicized. In part because of this publicity, the emphasis of the 1970s on controlling water and air pollution has been shifting slowly during the 1980s to the control of hazardous waste pollution. Despite this shifting emphasis, legislative and judicial systems have been slow to respond. Few remedies are available to real and imagined victims of toxic substances. From a legal point of view, there is little difference between exposure to low levels of radiation and low levels of toxic chemicals. Both instances fall under the broader domain of environmental law. Depending on the circumstances, one instance might provide legal precedent for the other. This chapter presents examples drawn from both areas in order to illustrate current issues.

This discussion is divided into four parts: (1) the common law tort theories that may be asserted when a plaintiff has suffered injury resulting from exposure to low-level radiation or other toxic substances; (2) the difficulties posed by the relief mechanisms rooted in traditional common law; (3) current federal legislation, along with its merits and shortcomings; and (4) solutions to the obstacles now faced by plaintiffs in attempting to recover their damages. Also discussed are suggested judicial and legislative solutions designed to remedy the damages caused to persons exposed to toxic wastes.

TRADITIONAL COMMON LAW THEORIES OF RECOVERY

A person who has suffered injury resulting from exposure to low-level radiation or toxic chemicals and who seeks legal recourse can proceed under several traditional common law tort theories. These theories — negligence, strict liability, trespass, and nuisance — are examined individually.

Negligence

Negligence has been defined as "the omission to do something which a reasonable man guided by those ordinary considerations which ordinarily regulate human affairs, would do, or the doing of something which a reasonable and prudent man would not do."[1] To prove a prima facie[2] case in negligence (i.e., "such as will prevail until contradicted and overcome by other evidence) the traditional formula requires that the plaintiff establish four elements: (1) existence of a duty to conform to a standard of conduct that protects others against unreasonable risks; (2) the defendant's failure to conform to that standard (i.e., a breach of duty); (3) a reasonably close causal connection between the defendant's conduct and the injury resulting to the plaintiff; and (4) the plaintiff's actual loss or injury.[3] These elements are discussed individually.

Existence of a Duty. In negligence cases, a duty may be defined as an obligation to which the law will give recognition and effect in order to conform to a particular standard of conduct toward another.[4] A plaintiff must first establish this duty to conform. Generally speaking, the duty imposed by law reflects both the magnitude of the risks involved and the existing state of knowledge concerning the activity at the time the activity was undertaken.[5]

Breach of Duty. After a plaintiff has established the existence of a duty, he or she must prove that the defendant breached that duty (i.e., the defendant failed to conform). In a case such as radiation exposure, the matter being litigated is of such a nature that a jury, on the basis of its common knowledge and experience, usually cannot determine whether a defendant has breached a duty. Expert testimony is required to establish the plaintiff's case.[6] The expert witness must testify that the defendant's conduct deviated from the standard of those similarly situated.

Causation. If the plaintiff is able to establish the first two elements — duty and breach of duty — he or she then must show injury as a direct and proximate cause of the defendant's conduct. To impose liability, the defendant's negligent act must be the cause of the plaintiff's injuries. This proof of causality involves two separate determinations: whether the defendant's conduct was the actual cause (or cause in fact) of the injury and whether it was the proximate (or legal) cause. In showing actual cause, the plaintiff must demonstrate that he or she would not have been injured had the defendant's act not occurred. In addition, it must also be determined whether such conduct was the proximate cause of the injury. Proximate cause, often referred to as legal causation, is essentially a question of policy as to whether the law will impose responsibility for the eventual consequences that might or might not have occurred as a result of the defendant's conduct.[7]

Damages. The fourth element that the plaintiff must show is an actual loss or damage resulting from the defendant's conduct. Negligent conduct in itself is not such an interference with the affairs of the world at large that there is any right to complain of it, or to be free from it, except in the event that some individual has suffered from the conduct.[8]

Strict Liability

The second theory under which a plaintiff can attempt to redress for damages suffered is strict liability. It should be noted that

> The hallmark of strict liability is . . . that it is imposed on lawful activities. The activities that qualify are those which entail extraordinary risk to others, either in the seriousness or the frequency of the harm threatened. Permission to conduct such activity is in effect made conditional on its absorbing the cost of the accidents it causes, as an appropriate item of its overhead cost.[9] In other words, strict liability is a theory of tort law that subjects a defendant to liability in some cases even though he has not departed in any way from a reasonable standard of care.[10]

Outside the products liability area, U.S. courts generally have held that defendants are subject to strict liability only when they engage in activities that are abnormally hazardous. Thus the critical question for a plaintiff asserting strict liability after exposure to radioactive or chemical waste is whether the disposition of the hazardous waste constitutes an abnormally dangerous activity.[11]

In determining whether an activity is abnormally hazardous, the following factors are to be considered[12]:

1. Existence of a high degree of risk of some harm to the person, land, or personal property of others
2. Likelihood that the harm that occurs will be great
3. Inability to eliminate the risk by the exercise of reasonable care
4. Extent to which the activity is not a matter of common usage
5. Inappropriateness of the activity in the location at which it is conducted
6. Extent to which the value of the activity to the community is outweighed by its dangerous attributes

Activities for which plaintiffs have been able to recover under the theory of strict liability include blasting, storage of oil near residences, percolating waters, fumigation with a dangerous chemical, and the emission of noxious gases from factories.[13] Under the theory of strict liability, the plaintiff is relieved from having to prove that the defendant failed to conform to a certain standard of conduct. However, the plaintiff must establish that the defendant was responsible for an abnormally dangerous activity.

Nuisance

In the common law theory of nuisance, private nuisance and public nuisance must be distinguished. A private nuisance is a civil wrong, being a disturbance of rights in land.[14] The remedy for the nuisance lies in the hands of the individual whose rights have been disturbed. On the other hand, a public or common nuisance is a type of "catch-all" criminal offense, emanating from an interference with the rights of the community at large.[14]

A plaintiff attempting to recover damages under the nuisance theory has to prove that a private nuisance exists that includes the following elements of the prima facie case: (1) act by the defendant; (2) a nontrespassory invasion of the plaintiff's interest; (3) intent, negligence, or strict liability; (4) substantial and unreasonable harm; and (5) causation.

In other words, the ability of a plaintiff to persuade a court to characterize the disposal of toxic wastes at a given location as a nuisance depends on whether the harm suffered constitutes a substantial and unreasonable interference with the use and enjoyment of the plaintiff's property.[15]

Trespass

Although trespass and nuisance developed historically as widely divergent concepts, they often are confused. Trespass connotes an invasion of the plaintiff's interest in the exclusive possession of his land, while nuisance refers to an interference with the use and enjoyment of the land.[16] Under this theory, the prima facie case that the plaintiff must prove includes the following elements: (1) an act by the defendant; (2) intent, negligence, or strict liability; (3) intrusion on the land; (4) plaintiff in possession or entitled to immediate possession; and (5) causation.

INADEQUACIES OF COMMON LAW REMEDIES

The lack of statutory remedies for those who have been harmed by radiation exposure necessitates reliance on common law remedies. It is extremely difficult, if not impossible, however, for plaintiffs to recover when asserting these common law theories. The three most frequently cited are inability (1) to prove the elements of a prima facie case, especially the causation element; (2)

to overcome the statute of limitation defense; and (3) to locate a culpable defendant. Other problems include lengthy delays, limited resources, and burdensome discovery.

Problems faced by a plaintiff in trying to prove a prima facie case of negligence, strict liability, trespass, or nuisance include the following. First, the elements of *negligence* are (1) existence of a duty; (2) breach of duty; (3) causation; and (4) injury. Often there is no problem in demonstrating an injury. However, the plaintiff might be unable to show duty or breach of duty because of inability to prove that the defendant had any obligation to take precautions other than those usually observed in the profession or industry, or because of failure to produce an expert witness who will testify that the defendant's activity was unreasonable at the time it occurred.[17]

Plaintiffs face a more formidable task in proving direct and proximate cause. In order to establish direct causation, the plaintiff must isolate the harm-causing agent, trace the pathway from the agent to the victim, and prove medically that the agent caused the injury or disease.[18] Because cancer and other diseases induced by radiation are indistinguishable from identical diseases induced by other causes such as heredity or other environmental hazards,[19] and because injury from radiation exposure can take decades to become manifest,[20] the proof of causation is frequently uncertain.

If a plaintiff is successful in establishing a causal connection, the next step is to prove further that the negligent act (e.g., the discharge of radioactive or chemical toxic waste) was a proximate, and not a remote, cause of the injuries. This requires a policy decision as to whether the defendant's liability should extend to the damages suffered by the plaintiff. In negligence cases, most courts have adopted a foreseeable test: a defendant is not liable for harm that could not be foreseen as resulting from his negligence.[21] Because of the long latency period involved with injuries resulting from low-level radiation exposures, the defendant might successfully defend the assertion that he or she was unable to foresee the plaintiff's damages.

Although the theory of strict liability might be the plaintiff's best common law remedy, there is still only a slight chance of recovery. As with negligence, the plaintiff must prove cause in fact. The difficulties with this proof have been discussed. Another obstacle the plaintiff faces under this theory is the categorization of the defendant's activity as ultrahazardous. The "ultrahazardous activity" test set forth above is extremely burdensome and difficult for the plaintiff to prove.

Trespass can offer relief only if the plaintiff can prove that an invasion has occurred as a result of the defendant's negligence, unusually dangerous activity, or intentional act. The difficulties of proving negligence or an abnormally dangerous activity discussed above also apply to trespass. Probably the biggest obstacle to proving trespass is the difficulty in characterizing the presence of radiation as a physical invasion of property. The theory of private nuisance offers little relief for personal injury, since it addresses property rights. A plaintiff choosing to assert an infringement of property rights must prove that the defendant's conduct was intentional, negligent, or abnormally dangerous. The difficulties encountered in proving these assertions have been discussed in relationship to the first three causes of action.

Another frequently encountered problem is the defendant's assertion of the statute of limitations. A statute of limitations is a "statute prescribing limitations to the right of action on certain described causes of action, that is, declaring that no suit shall be maintained on such causes of action unless brought within a specified period after the right accrued."[22] Most jurisdictions have a statute of limitations for tort claims of no more than 5 years. Because the statute begins to run when the tort is committed, recovery is traditionally prevented even if a plaintiff did not become aware of the injury until after the statutory period had ended. In low-level radiation exposure, for example, the statute of limitations would begin to run from the time the plaintiff was first exposed. This interpretation effectively precludes the plaintiff whose radiation injury lies dormant for 30 years.

Other major problems faced by a plaintiff are locating a culpable defendant and collecting a judgment. Because of the long latency period for injuries caused by toxic wastes and low-level radiation exposure, these problems are not uncommon. They exist where (1) a defendant cannot be found or identified; (2) the defendant is identified, but no longer exists as a legal entity (e.g., dissolved corporations); (3) the defendant's assets have been transferred to another legal entity; (4) the defendant is no longer in possession of the disposal property or radiation source; or (5) the defendant is insolvent and unable to provide compensation.[23]

INADEQUACIES OF FEDERAL LEGISLATION

Before the mid-1970s, most federal regulation of toxic substances was exercised by administrative agencies such as the Environmental Protection Agency (EPA) and Nuclear Regulatory Commission (NRC). This regulation was directed toward controlling the possibility of exposure rather than its consequences. The lack of federal regulation has been attributed to the belief held by Congress that problems of toxic substances were amenable to technical solutions developed by private industry and that management of such wastes was a state and local concern.[24] Although Congress did address the problem in 1976 when it passed the Resource Conservation and Recovery Act (RCRA),[25] compensation for victims of environmental pollution was not included in that piece of legislation. Despite this deficiency, RCRA has been touted as a systematic "cradle-to-grave" control of hazardous substances,[26] because it mandated that the EPA promulgate regulations, a listing of hazardous wastes, and the registration of generators, transporters, and disposal facilities for hazardous wastes.

In June 1979, legislation was initiated to establish a "superfund" of $1.6 billion to clean up hazardous waste dumps and emergency waste and oil spills.[27] After much change and debate, the House of Representatives accepted a compromise Senate bill signed by the president[28]:

> [The] Superfund Act provides a Hazardous Substances Response Trust Fund which is financed by chemical industry taxes and general revenues. It gives the President broad authority to respond to waste release incidents and to undertake cleanup efforts. Although Superfund will pay for response costs, remedial action and damage to natural resources caused by hazardous waste releases, fund representatives can sue responsible parties for reimbursement under a strict liability theory.

The deficiency of the Superfund Act is that it does not provide for compensation to victims. The state and federal governments that own or operate affected and damaged natural resources are the only third parties compensated by the Superfund.[29] Although the financial responsibility for hazardous wastes was placed on industry, the individual gained no statutory remedy for personal injuries under this Act.

The Superfund Act also provided for a separate postclosure liability fund in order to monitor and maintain sites permitted by the EPA and closed in accordance with EPA's closure standards. This liability fund covers only those facilities that have closed. This limitation is especially important, since EPA's insurance regulations apply only to active sites. In essence, the liability fund shifts the responsibility for long-term maintenance of hazardous waste disposal facilities from the private sector to the federal government, and the federal government assumes all responsibility for closed facilities, including property and personal injury to third parties.[30] It should be noted that the liability fund is more comprehensive than the Superfund because it covers personal and property damage, whereas the Superfund itself is restricted to clean up costs and natural resource damage.[31] This portion of the Act does help remedy the existing inadequacies of the common law. However, it is applicable only to closed facilities.

Recently, the EPA has promulgated regulations that require hazardous waste facilities to carry third-party liability coverage for the life of the facility under the authority of RCRA.[32] The net effect of the EPA's insurance regulations is to ensure the availability of funds for compensation of hazardous waste victims once a defendant is found liable.

Although some congressional members have attempted to draft laws to correct inadequacies of common law remedies and current legislation, Congress as a whole has been cautious in creating new remedies for private citizens for fear of overburdening industry.[33]

SUGGESTED SOLUTIONS TO COMMON LAW
AND FEDERAL LEGISLATIVE INADEQUACIES

It has been said that the goal of the legal system in this country is to provide a remedy to compensate an injured party for damages caused by another.[34] Arguments have been made that both common law and statutory remedies are inadequate for obtaining compensation for victims, and that the legal system is falling short of its goal. Legal authors have suggested various solutions to correct the problem. The suggestions fall into two categories: those mandated by statute and those prescribed by case law.

Proposed statutory changes include (1) methods to assist the plaintiff in establishing a prima facie case; (2) funds to provide compensation for damages once a defendant is proved liable; and (3) funds to provide compensation where the plaintiff is unable to prove that a specific defendant is liable.

To assist the plaintiff in establishing a prima facie case, it has been suggested that a federal cause of action on the basis of strict liability be enacted.[35] This shifting of accidental loss to the party most able to insure against the risk and bear the cost is a growing trend in tort law. The shift from fault to compensation analysis focuses on the goals of preventing the occurrence of injury and includes a consideration of cost shifting and risk spreading.[36] Another proposal is to relieve the plaintiff of the burden of proving negligence by lessening the burden of proof of medical causation. This could be done by providing that the injured party who was able to prove exposure to toxic wastes, for example, would satisfy the burden of proof "if a reasonable person would conclude . . . that injury or disease . . . is reasonably related to such discharge, release or disposal."[37] In other words, if the plaintiff could show a reasonable likelihood that injury was caused by exposure to a hazardous substance, he or she would benefit from a favorable presumption, and the defendant would have the burden of going forward. A proposed statutory provision for a rebuttable presumption of causation would go one step further in alleviating the plaintiff's problems of proving causation.[37] The burden of proof would be shifted to the defendant once the plaintiff had established a prima facie case.

Also recommended have been compensatory funds and insurance requirements designed to help victims find culpable defendants and collect judgments. While this alternative would not help the plaintiff establish a cause of action, it would ensure a source of compensation once damages had been awarded.[38]

A compensation system, including insurance in the form of third-party liability coverage or government-administered liability funds, has also been suggested. This system would permit victims to recover damages even if no defendant can be found or if a case cannot be proved under traditional bases of common law.[38] The suggested system is analogous to the compensation fund that was excluded from the Superfund legislation.

Proposed judicial changes include (1) a common law theory of strict liability; (2) acceptance of the statute of limitations discovery rule; and (3) implementation of risk benefit causation.

First, at least one author has suggested that the judiciary should address the rights of citizens by establishing a common law theory of strict liability for abnormally dangerous activities as a viable theory on which an individual may base a personal injury suit against an industry for hazardous waste poisoning.[39] The proposition that hazardous waste management should be deemed an abnormally dangerous activity by the courts is based on the precedent that strict liability has been found in situations analogous to hazardous waste cases.[40] A judicially imposed theory of strict liability is analogous to a statutorily imposed strict liability (see above).

Second, it has been suggested that the courts modify the statute of limitations in these cases. Traditionally, the statute begins to run when the damage occurs. This tradition leads to difficulties in cases of radiation exposure where the statute has run out by the time the victim has discovered the damage. Because courts could recognize that the intent behind the statute of limitations was not to deny justice for an entire group of injured citizens,[41] they could adopt the discovery rule for causes of action involving damage caused by radioactive or toxic wastes. The discovery rule "provides that in an appropriate case, a cause of action will be held not to accrue until the injured party discovers, or by the exercise of reasonable diligence and intelligence, should have discovered that he may have a basis for an actionable claim."[42]

Third, some authors believe that new approaches to causation such as risk benefit causation analysis should be implemented. The risk benefit approach represents one response to scientific uncertainty on causation questions in environmental lawsuits.[43] The courts have applied this approach in providing injunctive relief against a company discharging absestos fibers into the air.[44] The court stated that "when proof with certainty is impossible, the concept of harm, whether it be assessed at probability and consequences or risk and harm, necessarily must apply."[45]

Kuster[46] states

> that in implementing a risk benefit approach to causation analysis, the court would first make a threshold determination concerning the applicability of risk benefit analysis to the case before it. In making this threshold determination, the court would examine the nature of the scientific controversy, evaluating the degree of uncertainty presented. Where the uncertainty is unresolvable and touches on essential areas of the plaintiff's case, a strong case for lowering the burden on the causation issue would be made out; and risk benefit analysis would be deemed appropriate. The court would then proceed with a three-step analysis to assess the burden of proof. First, the seriousness of the plaintiff's injury would be weighed. Second, the court would examine the benefits to the community of the defendant's activities and the effects on those activities of imposing a damage

award on a company. In the third and final step, the court would balance this injury and benefit inquiries against the degree of uncertainty presented by the scientific information introduced into evidence. As the seriousness of the harm to plaintiff increases and the benefits of the defendant's activity become fewer, the less certain the need for proof of causation. On the basis of this balancing, the court would decide whether the evidence presented adequately shows a casual connection between defendant's actions and plaintiff's harm to enable the plaintiff to meet the burden of proving causation.

Fourth, a judicial shifting of the burden of proof has been suggested by Favish[47] to alleviate the plaintiff's problems of proving causation. Historically, courts have altered burdens of proof to reflect changing conditions or values; it is suggested that it is now time to alter the burden of proof for victims of toxic substances. In these cases, the plaintiff has provided as much circumstantial evidence of factual causation as could fairly be required under the circumstances. The courts then permitted a shift in the burden of proof on factual causation such that defendants were required to show their conduct did not, in fact, cause the plaintiff's injury.[47] It is proposed that the principles developed in these cases are applicable to persons exposed to radiation as well as to other toxic wastes.

CONCLUSION

Traditional common law actions of negligence, strict liability, trespass, and nuisance have been shown to be inadequate in providing relief to toxic waste victims. Current federal legislation has also been shown to have major shortcomings. Aware of these inadequacies, legal authorities have promulgated solutions that legislative and judicial bodies have the power to implement. Lawmaking bodies are also well acquainted with the present difficulties and have made small improvements by passing the Superfund Act. Nevertheless, many toxic waste victims remain without legal recourse and without compensation. These people are left to shoulder damages individually, which many think should more justly be borne by industry or government.

REFERENCES

1. *Black's Law Dictionary*, ed 5. West Publishing Co., St Paul, Minnesota 1979; 930.
2. *Black's Law Dictionary*, ed 5. West Publishing Co., St Paul, Minnesota 1979; 1071.
3. Prosser W: *Handbook of Law of Torts*, ed 4. West Publishing Co., St Paul, Minnesota 1971; 30.

4. Prosser W: Reference 3, p 53.
5. Prosser W: Reference 3, pp 28–34.
6. Aetna Insurance Company, Hellmuth, Obata and Kassabaum Inc., 392 F. 472, 478, 8th Cir. 1968.
7. Prosser W: Reference 3, p 42.
8. Prosser W: Reference 3, p 30.
9. Flemming J: *Law of Torts.* 1971; 273.
10. Prosser W: Reference 3, p 75.
11. Hurwitz W: Environmental health: An analysis of available and proposed remedies for victims of toxic waste contamination. *Am. J. Law Med.* 1981; 7.
12. Restatement (Second) of Torts. 1977; 502A.
13. Hurwitz W: Reference 11, p 77.
14. Prosser W: Reference 3, p 86.
15. Hurwitz W: Reference 11, p 84.
16. Prosser W: Reference 3, p 89.
17. Hurwitz W: Reference 11, p 66.
18. Meyer S: Compensating hazardous waste victims: RCRA insurance regulations and a not so "super" fund act. *Environmental Law.* 1981; 11:689.
19. Favish A: Radiation injury and the atomic veteran: Shifting the burden of proof on factual causation. *Hastings Law J* 1981.
20. Favish A: Reference 19, 32: 964.
21. Singer S: An analysis of common law and statutory remedies for hazardous waste injuries. *Rutgers Law J* 1980; 12:117.
22. *Black's Law Dictionary,* ed 5. West Publishing Co., St Paul, Minnesota 1979; 853.
23. Singer S: Reference 21, p 126.
24. Meyer S: Reference 18, p 693.
25. *The Resource Conservation and Recovery Act of 1976,* 1002, 42 USCA, 6901.
26. *EPA Issues RCRA's Cradle to Grave Hazardous Waste Rules, 1980.* 10 Environmental Law Report 10, 130.
27. S. 1341, H.R. 4571, 96th Congress first session, 1979.
28. Meyer S: Reference 18, p 699.
29. *Superfund Act of 1980,* Public Law 96-510, 107(a)(4)(c), (f), 94 Stat. 2767, 2781.
30. Meyer S: Reference 18, p 703.
31. *Superfund Act of 1980,* Public Law 96-510, 107(h), 111(j), 94 Stat. 2767, 2784, 2791.
32. 40 CFR 264. 147, 265. 147.
33. Bruno M: The development of a strict liability cause of action for personal injuries resulting from hazardous waste. *N Engl Law Rev* 1981; 16(3):543.
34. Meyer S: Reference 18, p 694.
35. Meyer S: Reference 18, p 712.
36. Bruno M: Reference 33, p 569.
37. Meyer S: Reference 18, p 717.
38. Meyer S: Reference 18, p 695.
39. Bruno M: Reference 33, p 571.
40. Restatement (Second) of Torts, 502A (1977).
41. Bruno M: Reference 33, p 571.

42. *Lopez vs Swyer*, 62 NJ, 267, 272; 300 A 2d 563, 1973.
43. Gelpe F: The uses of scientific information in environmental decisionmaking. *South Cal Law Rev* 1971; 48:371.
44. *Reserve Land Mining vs Environmental Protection Agency*, 514 F 2d 492, 8th Cir., 1975.
45. 514 F 2d 492 at 520.
46. Kuster B: Toxic substance contamination: The risk-benefit approach to causation analysis. *J Law Reform* 1980; 14 p 63.
47. Favish A: Reference 19, p 965.

21.

Health Effects in Residents of High Background Radiation Regions

Gerald P. Hanson

The phenomenon of areas of high natural radioactivity has been known to scientists since soon after the discovery of radioactivity by Henri Becquerel in 1896.[1] Pitchblende (uranium oxide ore) obtained from a mine at Joachimstal, Austria, was used by Marie Curie in her experiments concerning natural radioactivity, leading to the discovery of polonium and radium, and by Andre Debierne in the discovery of actinium. During the period 1910–1940, radium and radon were incorporated into medical cureall devices, and radium was injected into patients as therapy for a number of illnesses.[2] Colloidal thorium dioxide was introduced as a diagnostic contrast medium in 1928, and its use continued until about 1955.[3] Soon after the discovery of radioactivity, owners of spas promoted the healthful effects of their radioactive drinking water, and in old mines and areas of high natural radiation, the public has been encouraged to immerse themselves in the water and breathe the air as a cure for rheumatoid arthritis, endocrine and metabolic disorders, vascular diseases, and gerontic complaints.[4]

Although the health effects of radiation doses in occupationally exposed persons had received attention, it was not until the 1950s, when the atmospheric atom bomb tests of the United States and the Soviet Union had raised the level of environmental radioactivity, that the long-term effects of low-level radiation dosage became a matter of popular concern throughout the world. The United Nations Scientific Committee on the Effects of Atomic Radiation (UNSCEAR) was created, and the World Health Organization (WHO) appointed an expert committee to provide advice concerning radiation and human health. In its first report, the WHO expert committee identified several areas of high natural radiation where studies of the exposed population might possibly provide information concerning the effects of chronic low-level radiation dosage. This information, which was the best available in 1959, is shown in Table 1.[5]

193

TABLE 1.   AREAS OF HIGH NATURAL RADIATION IDENTIFIED BY THE WHO
EXPERT COMMITTEE ON RADIATION (1959) AS POSSIBLE RESEARCH SUBJECTS

Area	Average Natural Radiation Received, (mrad/year)	Exposed Population
Monazite region in India, parts of Kerala and Madras states	1300	80,000
Monazite region in Brazil, parts of states of Espirito Santo and Rio de Janeiro	500	50,000
Mineralized volcanic intrusives in Brazil, in states of Minas Gerais and Goiaz	1600	350
Primitive granitic, schistous, and sandstone areas of France	300	7,000,000

The WHO expert committee concluded that, on the basis of the available information, the Kerala area of India appeared to be the only one known at that time that might profitably be investigated. It was pointed out that there would be difficulties in conducting a study of the magnitude necessary to detect the small differences expected between the exposed and control populations. While the committee was fully aware of the desirability of obtaining meaningful information on the effects of chronic low-level doses, it pointedly stated that it was under no illusion regarding the probability that any investigation of high background radiation areas would demonstrate significant genetic changes. At approximately the same time that A.R. Gopal-Ayengar and K. Sundaram began their studies of the high natural radiation areas in India, scientists from the Catholic University (F.X. Roser and T.L. Cullen) and from the Federal University of Rio de Janeiro (C. Chagas and E. Penna Franca) began to study and report on the high natural radiation areas of Brazil. In addition to resources provided by the Brazilian National Research Council and the Nuclear Energy Commission, much valuable support was provided by Eisenbud and colleagues, the New York University Institute of Environmental Medicine and the U.S. Atomic Energy Commission, with the Pan American Health Organization helping to train national scientists and to coordinate the international efforts.

In 1973 the Pan American Health Organization took the initiative to bring together various international scientists, including the principal investigators for the studies in Brazil and India, for a meeting to exchange information, review progress, and discuss the needs for further research.[6] At this

Control Population	Available Health Statistics (Comments)
Similar ethnic groups in nearby areas	Some information could be obtained easily
Unknown	Information would be required
Unknown	Very little available
Remainder of French population	Information would be required

meeting it was concluded that, although the population groups being studied in Brazil and India were sizeable (India about 70,000 and Brazil about 6000), they were not large enough to measure subtle biologic effects over a wide range of chronic radiation doses. It was thought that an effort should be made to identify as many areas as possible in the world where population groups may be receiving doses comparable to the Indian and Brazilian study populations. The estimates at this time were a per-capita annual dose of 400 mrem in India and 700 mrem in Brazil. Tentative plans were made for convening an international meeting of investigators in the area of high natural radiation and a working definition was established for areas of chronic exposure which would qualify as "high natural radiation areas."

During the preparation for the International Symposium on Areas of High Natural Radioactivity, subsequently held at Pocos de Caldas, Brazil, in June 1975, and attended by 93 scientists from 16 countries, the working definition was modified slightly in deciding that only those areas that met one or more of the following criteria would be subject material:

1. The exposure rate from external sources over extended areas is >200 mR/year.
2. The long-lived α-activity ingested with the local diet (including water) is >50 pCi/day.
3. The radon-222 concentration of potable water is >5000 pCi/liter.
4. The radon-220 and radon-222 concentration of the atmosphere is >1 pCi/liter.[7]

At the International Symposium, the participants had a tendency to consider areas in which the natural radiation levels were more than three times the worldwide average as "elevated natural background areas," and those in which the natural levels were more than 10 times the worldwide average as "high background areas." Worldwide average values for radiation levels and doses are shown in Table 2, which is based on data from the 1977 UNSCEAR report.[8] In spite of variations in "normal" radiation levels, a large portion of the world population receives no more than two times the worldwide averages.

For example, the dose rate from cosmic radiation is 3.2 μrad/hr at sea level, increasing to 4.1, 6.2, and 9.8 μrad/hr at 1, 2, and 3 km above sea level, respectively. Although some large cities are located at high altitudes (e.g., Denver, Mexico City, Nairobi, and Teheran), the world average dose from cosmic radiation is very near the dose at sea level. In the case of terrestrial radiation, about 95 percent of the world population lives at an outdoor dose rate of 3–7 μrad/hr and at an indoor dose rate of 2–9 μrad/hr.

Areas of human exposure to high natural radiation levels have been identified on the basis of external dose or concentration of radionuclides in food or drinking water (see Tables 3 and 4). As shown in Table 3, the high external radiation levels reported are in Austria, Brazil, China, France, India, Iran, Italy, Madagascar, and Nigeria. When areas of high radionuclide intake are considered, as shown in Table 4, Finland and parts of the United States also enter into consideration.

On the basis of estimated average annual tissue doses and population sizes, it would appear that the most promising localities for health effects studies are Brazil and India, which have, in fact, been investigated; and perhaps the Helsinki area in Finland. The findings of various studies reported to date are presented below. Since details concerning methodology and quality control of data collection and processing were not provided, no judgment concerning the relative merit of the various studies has been attempted.

Austria.[4,9-14] An investigation of mortality in the Badgastein radioactive spa area in which nonradioactive spa areas with similar geographic and ecologic conditions were used as controls showed that cancer mortality was not higher and that longevity of the Badgastein population was not lower. A subsequent study of the risk of lung cancer led to the conclusion that any increase in the incidence of lung cancer would be difficult to observe because of the small sample size. Further studies showed that annual lung cancer incidence rates for Badgastein were not statistically different from the mean observed lung cancer incidence in the entire Province of Salzburg. However, it was observed that the persons who died of lung cancer had received a higher radiation dose than those who died of other causes.

Chromosome abberrations in the peripheral blood lymphocytes were also

TABLE 2. ESTIMATED WORLDWIDE AVERAGES OF RADIATION LEVELS AND WHOLE-BODY DOSES IN "NORMAL" RADIATION AREAS

Radiation Source *External Sources*	Absorbed Dose Rate in Air	Annual Dose, (mrad)
Cosmic rays (at sea level)	3.2 μrad/hr	28
Terrestrial radiation		
Outdoors	4.5 μrad/hr	
Indoors	5.3 μrad/hr	32 (combined outdoors plus indoors)

Radiation Source *Internal Sources*	Intakes or Concentrations	Annual Dose, (mrad)
Cosmogenic radionuclides (^{14}C, ^3H, ^7Be, ^{22}Na)	—	1.3
Primordial radionuclides		
Potassium–40	1600 pCi/kg concentration in tissue	17
Rubidium–87	230 pCi/kg concentration in tissue	0.4
Radium–226	1 pCi/day intake	0.03 (0.7 to bone lining cells)
Radium–228	1 pCi/day intake	0.06 (1.1 to bone-lining cells)
Lead–210	3 pCi/day intake	0.0006
Polonium–210	3 pCi/day intake	0.6 (3.4 to bone-lining cells)
Radon–222		
Outdoor air	0.1 pCi/liter concentration in continental air	1 (lung) 0.007 (gonads)
Indoor air	0.1–1 pCi/liter concentration	30 (lung) 0.2 (gonads)
Radon–220 (thoron)		
Outdoor air	0.001 pCi/liter concentration	0.1 (lung) 0.0002 (gonads)
Indoor air	0.01 pCi/liter concentration	4 (lung) 0.008 (gonads)
Thorium–232	0.1 pCi/day intake	0.04 (lung) 0.004 (gonads)
Uranium–238	0.4 pCi/day intake	0.04 (lung) 0.04 (gonads)

Estimated total external and internal annual whole-body dose, rounded to nearest whole number: 79 mrad

TABLE 3. AREAS OF HUMAN EXPOSURE TO HIGH EXTERNAL RADIATION LEVELS

Area	Absorbed Dose rate in air (μ rad/hr) [a]	Population	Average Annual Absorbed Dose in Tissue (rad).
Austria			
Badgastein	8–29	6500	0.07–0.2
Brazil			
Monazite area			
Guarapari	100–200 in streets (2000 peak on beach)	12,000	0.55 (range 0.09–2.8)
Meaipe	130 (peak 1000)	300	—
Cumuruxatiba	50	—	—
Volcanic intrusive			
area Araxá-Tapira	400	350	—
China			
Guangdon Province (Dong-anling and Tongyou)	20–27	73,000	0.2
France			
Languedoc–Roussillon	1–30 (peak 1000)	—	—
India			
Kerala state	150	70,000	0.4–0.5
Iran			
Ramsar	80–5500	2000	1.5
Italy			
Lazio and Campania	—	—	—
Madagascar	—	—	—
Nigeria	—	—	—

[a] 200 mrem/year = 23 μrad/hr.

studied for population groups of Badgastein, including the inhabitants of the area, spa-house personnel, and doctors and supporting staff working in the thermal gallery and the treatment house. The study included an analysis of 30,770 cells from 122 persons for aneuploid and polyploid cells, morphologically abnormal chromosomes, and chromatid and chromosome aberrations (gaps, breaks, exchanges, fragments, interstitial deletions, and dicentrics). No rings were observed. Since the chromosome aberration frequency was found to be age-dependent, the results were normalized to an age of 50 years.

TABLE 4. AREAS OF HIGH CONCENTRATION OR HIGH HUMAN INTAKE OF RADIONUCLIDES

Area	Radionuclide	Daily Intake or Concentration	Population	Dose to Tissue
Austria				
Badgastein	Radion-222	Air concentration of 0.8–3000 pCi/liter	6500	Bronchioles, 2–320 rem/year
Brazil				
Volcanic intrusive area, Araxa-Tapira	Radium-226 Radium-228	20–40 pCi/day 120–240 pCi/day	200	—
Finland				
Helsinki	Radon-222	Average drinking water concentration of 17,000 pCi/liter	150,000	Lungs (11 rem/year
India				
Kerala state	Gross alpha Radium-228	215 pCi/day 160 pCi/day	70,000	—
United States				
Illinois, Iowa	Radium-226	Concentration in drinking water 3–80 pCi/liter	900,000	—
Maine	Radon-222	Concentration in drinking water 10,000–60,000 pCi/liter	—	
Texas	Radium-226	Concentration in drinking water 10–15 pCi/liter	1000	—
	Radon-220	Concentration in drinking water 1000–8000 pCi/liter	1000	—

The dose effect curve for combined α and γ irradiation for all types of aberrations was observed to rise sharply to an annual dose of 200–300 mrad which was attributed mainly to continuous background γ radiation. At doses above 300 mrad per year, attributed to additional α irradiation, the dose-response curve reached a plateau.

The data were analyzed further by dividing the population into persons who only received "normal" background irradiation (mainly γ with a very small α component) and persons who receive a higher α dose in addition to the γ dose. This analysis showed a sharply rising dose-response curve for the group subjected only to "normal" background irradiation. For those subjected to a higher α irradiation component, the response was less dose dependent; and for the group receiving the highest α dose (higher than 100 mrad per month) the response curve reached a peak and even turned downward for two-break events. These results were unexpected, and the authors postulated that the explanation could be the activity of repair enzymes that were regulated by a threshold phenomenon.

Brazil.[7] Since the population size is small and there is a paucity of sufficient medical records, no mortality or morbidity studies have been made in Brazil. A study of somatic chromosomal aberrations in peripheral lymphocytes was conducted in the Guarapari area (mean annual external radiation level 640 mr, with a range of 100-3200 mr) with 13,242 cells from 202 persons. The control group consisted of residents of a village with a similar socioeconomic level and a normal background radiation level (9001 cells in 147 persons were analyzed). There was no significant difference in the number of aneuploid cells or chromatid aberrations, neither of which was considered radiation-induced damage. A significant increase in the total number of chromosomal breaks (a deletion was counted as one break and a dicentric was counted as two breaks) was observed in the Guarapari residents ($p<0.05$). This was interpreted as an effect of the higher level of natural radiation in the Guarapari area and is thought to be attributable to inhalation of the decay products of thoron (lead-212 and bismuth-212) rather than to higher external radiation levels. This hypothesis was supported by a cytogenetic survey of workers exposed to much higher levels of thoron daughters in a nearby monazite ore mill, and in whom a positive correlation was found between levels of airborne lead-212 and bismuth-212 and chromosomal aberrations.

China.[15] During 1972-1975 in the Dong-anling and Tongyou areas of Guangdong Province, a population of about 73,000 whose families had been living in an elevated radiation level for many generations (90.6 percent of the study group families had lived in the area for six or more generations) was compared with a control group of 77,000 persons living in nearby areas (Sanhe) having similar geographic, socioeconomic, and ethnic characteristics. The study group received an average annual dose of about 200 mrad to the whole body from external radiation and the control group received about 70 mrad; the internal dose contributions to the whole body were about 35 and 24 mrad, respectively.

A clinical examination of infants and children less than 12 years of age (3,504 from the study group and 3,170 controls) for 31 kinds of hereditary diseases and congenital deformaties showed no statistically significant difference. The incidence of Down's syndrome was higher in the study group, with a frequency of 1.71:1000 versus zero in the control group. However, because of the small size of the population, the researchers were concerned about the significance, realizing that further investigation was necessary.

Measurements of children less than 12 years of age (3,239 from the study group and 2,991 controls) for height, weight, and head circumference showed no significant differences in growth and development. The spontaneous abortion rate between 1963 and 1975 of 73.9:1,000 for the study group and 72.5:1,000 for the control group showed no difference between the study group (1,551 women and 3,896 pregnancies) and the control group (1,716 women and 3,062 pregnancies).

In 1975 the frequency of malignancies observed through clinical examination was not significantly different between the study group (20,154 persons) and the control group (21,235 persons). A retrospective survey of cancer mortality covering the period 1970–1974 showed no significant difference between the study group (96,533 person-years) and the control group (122,554 person-years) for such malignancies as breast, cervix, esophagus, intestine, liver, lung, and nasopharynx.

Cytogenetic studies were done of peripheral lymphocytes; no significant difference between inhabitants of the high background radiation areas and the control area was found in the frequencies of chromatid or chromosomal aberrations.

India.[7] One group of scientists from the Bhabha Atomic Research Center carried out a detailed demographic survey of the population (70,000 persons in 13,355 households) living in the high natural radiation background area of Kerala state. Since the high background area is essentially a strip of land about 55 km long and 0.5 km wide interrupted by areas of normal background radiation, the control population was from these normal areas with similar socioeconomic and religious characteristics. On the basis of a sampling of 20 percent of the households, about 16,600 of the 70,000 persons living in the area were estimated to be receiving a dose in excess of 0.5 rad/year, with the per-capita dose about 0.4 rad/year. Analysis of the data failed to show any statistically significant difference for groups receiving different levels of radiation in fertility index, sex ratio among offspring, infant mortality rate, pregnancy terminations, multiple births, or gross congenital abnormalities. The researchers concluded that the variables studied were not sensitive enough to modification by radiation to show any statistically significant differences. They did observe, however, that a group that received more than 20 times the normal background radiation exposure had the lowest value of fertility index and the highest value of infant mortality.

Another group of researchers, from the All-India Institute of Medical Sciences, while studying the enlargement of the thyroid gland and finding no difference in the histologic characteristics of goiter between a population living in the high natural radiation area and a control group living in an area of normal background radiation, did observe a higher frequency of Down's syndrome. Twelve cases were observed in the study population of about 12,000 persons as compared with no cases of Down's syndrome in the control population of about 6000 persons. Although this frequency of Down's syndrome (1:1000) is one of the highest observed worldwide, it was mentioned during the discussion of these findings that a frequency of about 1:800 had been observed in a population group living in New Delhi, where radiation levels are normal.

A complicating factor in this study is that no radiation dosimetric data were presented; also, it has been shown that radiation exposure is highly variable in monazite areas, so that an individual living near the monazite sands does not necessarily receive a high radiation dose. Additional observations by this group of researchers included a higher frequency of severe mental abnormality of genetic origin (23 cases in the study population versus four cases in the control) and a higher frequency of limb malformations (three cases in the study population versus zero in the control).

Further cytogenetic studies of chromosomal aberrations in cultured whole blood by the group from the All-India Institute of Medical Sciences gave the results shown in Table 5. The number of chromosomal aberrations in all four study groups differed significantly from findings in the control group ($p<0.001$). The most common types of chromosomal aberrations were deletions and acentric fragments (mean 2.5, with a range of 1.4–3.2 per 100 cells), and the number of dicentrics and rings was low (mean 0.6 with a range of 0.4–1.2 per 100 cells). The researchers suggest that the chronic low-level radiation is causing genetic damage in the population.

United States (Midwest Environmental Health Study).[7,16] In 1962 a retrospective study of approximately 900,000 residents of the states of Illinois and

TABLE 5.   RESULTS OF CYTOGENIC STUDIES IN THE HIGH BACKGROUND AREA OF KERALA STATE

Population Group	Number of Persons Studied	Chromosomal Aberrations per 100 Cells
Control (Purrakade-Punnapura)	39	0.2
High radiation area	46	1.9
Workers in Monazite industry (Manavalakurichi)	17	3.1
Patients with Down's syndrome	—	3.5
Parents of patients with Down's syndrome	—	3.6

Iowa was initiated to determine whether this population living in communities with a high radium-226 concentration in drinking water (weighted mean of 4.7 pCi/liter), and with approximately equal levels of radium-224 and radium-228, exhibited health effects at a higher rate than did a control population from similar communities with a radium-226 concentration of <1 pCi/liter in their water supplies. The overall age-adjusted and sex-adjusted mortality rates for deaths due to malignant neoplasms involving bone were greater in the communities with high radium-226 levels in the water supplies than in control communities ($p = 0.08$). When age-specific mortality rates for malignant neoplasms involving bone were calculated for the specific age groups of 20–29 and 60–69, the mortality rates were greater in the population exposed to higher radium-226 levels and were considered significant, with p values of 0.01 and 0.07, respectively. In four of the remaining seven age groups, the mortality rates were higher in the exposed population than in the control; however, these differences were not considered significant.

Although there is some concern over the findings (see below), the researchers concluded that "the adjusted mortality rates based on deaths coded to malignant neoplasms involving bone were consistently and sometimes significantly higher in the exposed population than in the control."[7]

Concern over the validity of the findings involves the following statistical correlations:

1. Two neighboring states (Wisconsin and Missouri), portions of which have water with high radium-226 levels, but apparently not in public drinking water supplies, had higher mortality rates from malignant neoplasms involving bone as compared with the control population, but lower than in the exposed population.

2. The mortality rate from malignant neoplasms involving bone in the city of Chicago, Illinois, which obtains its drinking water from Lake Michigan, with a radium-226 content of only 0.03 pCi/liter, was higher than in the exposed population.

3. Apparently, the crude mortality rate from malignant neoplasms involving bone (deaths per 100,000 per year) decreased during the period of the study from 1.6 in 1950 to about 0.95 in 1962, with this decrease being entirely in the age group of 30 and over.

4. If the study had used the key words "sarcoma" or "Ewing's tumor" in reviewing death certificates, rather than the broader concept of malignant neoplasms involving bone, a clearer indication of radiation-induced neoplasms would be expected. However, when the analysis was made on this basis, no significant difference was observed in the mortality rates between the exposed and control populations.

Additional complicating factors, which have led other scientists to conclude that no health effect could be attributed to high radium-226 levels in
drinking water, are the following:

1. Since water-softening units remove radium, some households in the
    exposed area might have consumed little radium.
2. Since the population is mobile, it is very difficult to determine how
    long any kind of water might have been consumed.
3. Since bottled sources of liquid are used by much of the population, it
    is difficult to know the exact origin of the water that was consumed.

United States (Drinking Water and Cancer Incidence In Iowa).[17,18] Using
statewide Iowa cancer incidence data for the years 1969-1971 and 1973-1978,
age-adjusted, sex-specific rates for 6 cancer sites (bladder, breast, colon,
lung, prostate, rectum) were calculated for groups of municipalities and were
compared with the levels of radium 226 in the drinking water. The following
criteria were used for selecting municipalities to be included in the study:

a. population of 1,000-10,000;
b. a public water supply derived solely from wells more than 152 meters
    deep;
c. the public water supply was not softened.

The 28 municipalities which qualified for inclusion in the study were placed
in 3 groups according to radium 226 content of 0-2, 2-4.9, and greater than
5 pCi/liter. The rates of lung cancer for males were observed to increase with
radium 226 levels, and the relative risk for those in the highest group was 1.68
times that of the lowest group. The test of the hypothesis that the rate of male
lung cancer was the same for all 3 groups of municipalities showed a significant difference ($p < .002$). The test of the hypothesis for female breast cancer
showed the difference was not as significant ($p = 0.07$). When the municipalities were divided into two groups (those with less than $3pCi\ l^{-1}$ and those
with greater than $3pCi\ l^{-1}$), it was found that age-specific lung cancer rates
for males of all age groupings were higher for those municipalities with
greater than $3pCi\ l^{-1}$ of radium 226. When smoking habits were investigated,
it was observed that there was no parallel between geographic differences in
smoking and differences in radium levels of water supplies, and it was accepted that smoking patterns were similar. Other potential explanatory
variables examined by multiple regression analysis were: median income,
occupation (e.g., % of manufacturing and percent of agricultural workers)
and fluoride level of the water. After these variables were entered, a significant relationship still remained between radium 226 level and male lung
cancer ($p = 0.028$). The authors noted that geographic mobility during the

onset of disease and the usage of home water softeners (which are installed in about 42% of Iowa homes) would both tend to reduce the population at risk. It was suggested that radium 226 measurements may be a surrogate for radon 222 and other radioactive elements, and that while definitive relationships could not be established, more detailed studies should be considered.

The data concerning the studies of chronic exposure of human populations to higher than normal levels of natural background radiation can be summarized as follows:

1. Effects (aberrations) have been observed in the chromosomes.
2. Down's syndrome has been observed and could be related to radiation exposure.
3. Malignant neoplasms related to bone apparently correspond to high concentrations of radium-226 in drinking water. There is concern about the validity of this conclusion. However, the same complicating factors cited as causing concern about the findings could very well be operating to reduce the number of malignant neoplasms that might otherwise have been observed (e.g., water softening, population mobility, and intake of liquids from outside the area). In addition, when the population was divided into just two age groups (above and below 30 years of age), the mortality for the population below age 30, with high radium-226 content in their drinking water, was higher than for the control population ($p = 0.10$). This finding agrees with theoretical concepts postulated by Pochin[19] concerning the optimum age of populations to be studied for evidence of fatal malignancies caused by radiation.
4. Although various researchers have looked for them, effects have not been demonstrated regarding cancer mortality (other than malignant neoplasms involving bone), gross congenital abnormalities, fertility index, growth and development, hereditary disease (other than the possibility of Down's syndrome), infant mortality, longevity, multiple births, sex ratio, or spontaneous abortion rate.

The fact that these effects have not been demonstrated could be attributable to any of several factors:

1. The normal frequency in the population might be so high that the excess in the population exposed to the higher radiation levels cannot be determined in the relatively small sizes of the populations investigated.
2. Insufficient discipline might have been maintained over the experimental observations, and errors could have been made in obtaining the data.
3. The health effects might not occur at the levels of radiation to which

TABLE 6. RELATIVE RISK IN A COHORT STUDY THAT CAN BE DETECTED WITH
A POWER OF −0.9 AND AN α −0.5 (One-Tailed)[a]

Person-years of Observation per Group	0.5	1	2	4
100	>1000	>1000	>1000	>1000
250	>1000	>1000	>1000	839
500	>1000	>1000	849	426
1,000	>1000	854	429	216
2,000	860	430	216	110
4,000	432	217	110	56
6,000	289	146	74	39
8,000	218	110	56	30
10,000	175	89	46	24
15,000	118	60	31	17
20,000	89	46	24	13
30,000	60	31	17	9.8
40,000	46	24	13	7.9
50,000	37	20	11	6.8
70,000	27	15	8.7	5.4
100,000	20	11	6.8	4.4
200,000	11	6.8	4.4	3.1
500,000	5.9	3.9	2.8	2.2
750,000	4.6	3.2	2.4	1.91
1,000,000	3.9	2.8	2.2	1.77
5,000,000	2.0	1.68	1.46	1.31
10,000,000	1.68	1.46	1.32	1.22

[a] Figures are based on the calculations of Dr. R. E. Shore, New York University
is that of Schlesselman J: Sample size requirements in cohort and case

the populations have been exposed; there might be a level of radiation below which the effect is either not induced or is repaired after it
is induced.

Regarding cancer risks, the issue of statistically valid conclusions has
been discussed by Land[20] who has given the following example based on the
assumption that excess risk is proportional to radiation dose. If a population
of 1000 were needed to determine the effect of 100 rad, then for lower doses
the following numbers would be required:

       10 rad   100,000 population
        1 rad   10,000,000 population

One of Land's contentions is that in view of the lack of resources for adequate studies of populations exposed to low levels of radiation, considerable
risk is involved in trying to do the studies anyway, since misleading results

Annual Incidence in Control Group per 100,000							
8	12	16	24	32	48	64	100
>1000	675	507	339	255	171	129	84
421	282	212	142	107	73	55	36
215	144	109	73	56	38	29	20
109	74	56	38	29	21	16	11
56	38	30	21	16	12	9.3	6.8
30	21	16	12	9.3	6.9	5.7	4.4
21	15	12	8.5	7.0	5.3	4.5	3.5
16	12	9.3	7.0	5.7	4.5	3.8	3.1
13	9.8	7.9	6.0	5.0	4.0	3.4	2.8
9.8	7.3	6.0	4.7	4.0	3.2	2.9	2.4
7.9	6.0	5.0	4.0	3.4	2.9	2.5	2.2
6.0	4.7	4.0	3.2	2.9	2.4.	2.2	1.91
5.0	4.0	3.4	2.9	2.5	2.2	2.0	1.77
4.4	3.5	3.1	2.6	2.3	2.0	1.9	1.68
3.7	3.0	2.7	2.3	2.1	1.85	1.72	1.56
3.1	2.6	2.3	2.0	1.88	1.69	1.59	1.46
2.3	2.0	1.88	1.69	1.59	1.47	1.40	1.32
1.77	1.61	1.52	1.42	1.36	1.29	1.23	1.19
1.61	1.49	1.42	1.33	1.29	1.23	1.20	1.16
1.52	1.42	1.36	1.29	1.25	1.20	1.17	1.14
1.22	1.18	1.15	1.12	1.10	1.08	1.07	1.06
1.15	1.12	1.11	1.09	1.07	1.06	1.05	1.04

Medical Center Institute of Environmental Medicine. The basic formula
control studies of disease. Am J Epidemiol 1974; 99: 381–384.

could be obtained that would derive undue credibility simply because of the effort expended.

The statistical issue of the matter of the population size required for cohort studies of radiation effects is illustrated in Table 6.

For example, let us assume a normal incidence of disease in the control group of 12:100,000/year and an incidence in the exposed population (during the duration of the study) twice that of the controls. In that case, both the control and the exposed populations would have to have 200,000 person-years of observation in order to achieve a 90 percent chance of finding a statistically significant difference, if one actually exists, and only a 5 percent chance that a significant difference would be claimed if one does not really exist.

In performing a feasibility study for the Nuclear Regulatory Commission, in response to a mandate from the U.S. Congress for an evaluation to determine whether more epidemiologic research should be carried out to answer some of the controversy about the effects of low doses of radiation, Dreyer and her colleagues[22] concluded that in view of the uncertainties involved, "no single population can securely provide enough information to distinguish the absence of effects from small effects at low doses." To overcome this difficulty, the pooling of data from studies of different groups was suggested. For their study, Dreyer and associates defined "low dose" as a single dose of $\leqslant$ 5 rem to the whole body or a chronic dose accumulated at the rate of $\leqslant$ 5 rem/year; these workers included both populations that were occupationally exposed as well as those exposed to special environmental radiation conditions.

In a report to the U.S. Congress, the Government Accounting Office[23] concluded that "there is as yet no way to determine precisely the cancer risks of low-level ionizing radiation exposure, and it is unlikely that this question will be resolved soon."

The prognosis for fruitful epidemiologic studies of populations exposed to high natural radiation levels is not very good. However, bearing in mind the difficulties involved in attempting to extrapolate effects observed at high doses and high-dose rates, or in animal studies, to chronic low-level doses received by humans, the recommendations made during the International Symposium on Areas of High Natural Radioactivity in Brazil are listed below:

1. The World Health Organization (WHO), International Atomic Energy Agency (IAEA), and the Food and Agricultural Organization (FAO) should encourage documentation of radioactive anomalies and the extent of exposure of indigenous human populations. These agencies of the United Nations should also assist in establishing a worldwide system for comparing measurement and analytic techniques. This is particularly necessary for analytic procedures involving the heavy radionuclides, but it is desirable for external radiation measurements as well.

2. The data on human exposure to thoron and radon in buildings are inadequate; systematic measurements should be encouraged.

3. There is a need for long-term measurements of the dose to the lung from the radon daughters. The dose should be expressed as rem to the basal cells of the bronchial epithelium.

4. WHO, in collaboration with the IAEA, should offer assistance to developing nations that wish to assess the extent of the exposure of their populations to natural radioactivity.

5. All public water supplies derived from aquifers in sandstone or fractured granitic rock or aquifers in contact with black shales should be sampled for radium-226. If the concentration is $>$ 1 pCi/liter, additional measurements should be made for radium-228, lead-210, and polonium-210.

6. The epidemiologic work in Kerala state and Brazil should be continued. A firm negative finding would be useful, and there is the possibility that with development of new techniques some new unanticipated effects will be observed.

7. WHO-FAO should communicate with departments of agriculture in member states requesting that they provide information on the extent of farmland known to be fertilized naturally with uraniferous phosphates.

8. WHO-FAO should request member states to identify locations of public water supplies known to be derived from aquifers in contact with sandstone, fractured granite, or black shales.

9. The question of whether radiation resistance has developed among indigenous flora and fauna in areas near radioactive anomalies should be investigated.

Taking into account the scarcity of resources, it is understandable that some recommendations were neither feasible nor of sufficient priority to warrant action.

However, in view of current knowledge, several of these recommendations merit further consideration (e.g., items 2, 3, and 6, at least as far as Kerala state is concerned). With regard to recommendations 2 and 3, it is noteworthy that in a nationwide sampling of Canadian homes carried out in the summer months of 1977 and 1978, it was found that about 36 percent of the homes had radon concentrations > 1 pCi. In homes with basements, samples were taken there, where ventilation is poor and radon tends to accumulate there; in homes without a basement, the sample was taken at ground level.[24] Extension of this work has now included over 14000 homes in 18 Canadian cities with a total population of 11 million inhabitants, and the relationship between lung cancer mortality and radon daughter concentrations has been investigated while controlling for smoking habits.[25] The results show no association between radon daughter concentrations and lung cancer mortality, with or without the adjustment for smoking habits, and suggest that any effect of radon-daughter exposure on lung cancer mortality must be small in comparison to the effect of smoking.

Other surveys carried out in Canada, Sweden, and the United States have indicated that sizeable population groups may be exposed to average radon concentrations in the range of 2–10 pCi/liter and that in some locations (Sweden and Eastern Pennsylvania) more than 10 percent of the study population might be exposed to concentrations > 20 pCi/liter.[26] Building materials, underlying soil and rocks, and well water have been identified as sources of radon in homes with high concentrations.[27] In addition, efforts to conserve energy by tightly sealing houses, and thereby reducing ventilation, have resulted in higher radon levels.

The findings concerning exposure to radon in homes have caused a dilemma. If a philosophy similar to that concerning human-induced radiation sources were followed, requiring the limitation of radiation dose to population groups to a small fraction (e.g., one-thirtieth to one-tenth the occupational dose limit), the construction of a very large number of dwellings would have to be altered.[28] If this dose limit for population groups were increased to one-fourth the occupational limit, it would still require the altered construction of about 4 percent of houses in the United States, with the corresponding psychological and financial stresses for their owners. In terms of lung cancer, the situation would be as shown in Table 7.

According to calculations by Harley,[20] if the population exposure were limited to the indicated fractions of the occupational limit, the corresponding yearly reductions in lung cancer incidence would be as shown below:

1/2 occupational limit =   600 lung cancer cases eliminated
1/4 occupational limit = 1500 lung cancer cases eliminated
1/8 occupational limit = 3000 lung cancer cases eliminated

The alterations that might be required could be very costly; hence a balance between risk reduction and cost must be achieved.

Having traced the development of studies of high background radiation regions from the 1950s to the 1980s, it might be observed that a clear quantitative conception of the risk of low-level exposure to radiation, on the basis of epidemiologic observations in human populations, is as urgently needed as ever. The following observation attributed to the early Brazilian proponents of epidemiologic studies in high natural radiation areas[7] is as valid today as it was nearly 30 years ago:

Nature has been performing experiments for us for centuries. We need only the intelligence to ask of her the right questions.

TABLE 7.   ESTIMATED ANNUAL RISK OF DEATH FROM LUNG CANCER FOR VALUES OF RADON DAUGHTER EXPOSURE LIMITATION

Radon Daughter Exposure Limitation (Expressed as Fraction of Occupational Limit of 4 WLMY^{-1})	Risk of Death from Lung Cancer[a] (Deaths per Year Per Million Persons Exposed)
1/20[b]	40
1/10	80
1/8	100
1/4	200
1/2	400
1	800

[a]After age 40.
[b]Estimated average natural background in the United States.

REFERENCES

1. Jenkins EN: *Radioactivity, A Science in Its Historical and Social Context.* Liverpool, Wykeham Publications, 1979.
2. Eisenbud M: *Environmental Radioactivity.* New York, Academic Press, 1973.
3. WHO: Report of the WHO Scientific Group on the Long-Term Effects of Radium and Thorium in Man, Geneva, September 12-16, 1977.
4. Pohl-Rüling J, Scherminzky F: The natural radiation environment of Badgastein, Austria and its biological effects. Presented at the Symposium The Natural Radiation Environment II. Houston, Texas, August 7-11, 1972.
5. WHO: Effect of Radiation on Human Heredity: Investigation of Areas of High Natural Radiation, Technical Report Series No 166. Geneva, World Health Organization, 1959.
6. Pan American Health Organization: Areas of High Natural Radioactivity (Planning Session) Washington DC, December 18-20, 1973.
7. Brazilian Academy of Sciences: International Symposium on Areas of High Natural Radioactivity. Pocos de Caldas, Brazil, June 16-20, 1975. Rio de Janeiro, Academia Brasileira de Ciencias, 1977.
8. United Nations Scientific Committee on the Effects of Atomic Radiation, 1977 Report to the General Assembly, with Annexes. Sources and Effects of Ionizing Radiation. New York, United Nations, 1977.
9. Pohl-Rüling J: Final Report. Chromosome Aberrations in the Peripheral Blood Lymphocytes of People Living or Working in Areas of Higher Atmospheric Concentration of Natural Radon-222 and Its Daughters in Badgastein, Austria. International Atomic Energy Agency Contact No. 791/RB, 791/R,1RB, 791/R2/RB, Salzburg, December 1973.
10. Steinhäusler F: Long-Term Investigations in Austria of Environmental Natural Sources of Ionizing Radiation and Their Impact on Man. Ber Nat Med Ver Salzburg, Band 6, 1982: 7-50.
11. Pohl-Rüling J, Pohl E, et al.: Radiation Risk in Radon Spas. Medecine Biologie Environment (in press).
12. Pohl-Rüling J: The Dose-Effect Relationship of Chromosome Aberrations to Alpha and Gamma Irradiation in a Population Subjected to an Increased Burden of Natural Radioactivity. Radiat Res 1979; 80: 61-81.
13. Pohl-Rüling J: Biological Effects in a Population Living in an Elevated Natural Radioactive Environment. Nordic Society For Radiation Protection Meeting on Natural Radioactivity in Our Environment, Geilo, Norway, 6-9 January 1980.
14. Pohl-Rüling J: An Epidemiological Study on Chromosome Aberrations in a Radon Spa. Proceedings, Radon Specialist Meeting, Rome, Italy, March 1980 (in press).
15. High Background Research Group: Health survey in high background radiation areas in China. *Science* 1980; 209:877-880.
16. Petersen NJ, Samuels LD, et al.: An Epidemiologic Approach to Low-Level Radium 226 Exposure. Public Health Rep 1966; 81 (9): 805-814.
17. Bean J, Isacson P, et al.: Drinking Water and Cancer Incidence in Iowa, I. Trends and Incidence by Source of Drinking Water and Size of Municipality. Am J Epidemiol 1982; 116(6): 912-923.
18. Bean J, Isacson P, et al.: Drinking Water and Cancer Incidence in Iowa, II.

Radioactivity in Drinking Water. Am J Epidemiol 1982; 116(6): 924-932.

19. Pochin EE: Problems involved in detecting increased malignancy rates in areas of high natural radiation background. *Health Phys* 1976; 31:148-151.

20. Land CE: Estimating cancer risks from low doses of ionizing radiation. *Science* 1980; 209:1197-1203.

21. Schlesselman J: Sample size requirements in cohort and case control studies of disease. *Am J Epidemiol* 1974; 99:381-384.

22. Dreyer N, Loughlin JE, Friedlander ER, et al: Choosing populations to study the health effects of low-dose ionizing radiation. *Am J Publ Health* 71:1247-1252.

23. GAO: Problems in Assessing the Cancer Risks of Low-Level Ionizing Radiation Exposure. Report to the Congress of the United States by the Comptroller General, January 1981.

24. McGregor RG, Vasudev P, Letourneau EG, et al: Background concentrations of radon and radon daughters in Canadian homes. *Health Phys* 1980; 39: 285-289.

25. Letourneau E: Radiation Protection in Canada. Scientific Briefing Session. Eighteenth Annual Meeting of the National Council on Radiation Protection and Measurements, Washington DC, NCRP, 1982.

26. Oswald RA, Alter HW, Gingrich JE: Indoor Radon Measurements with Track Etch Detectors. Twenty-Seventh Annual Meeting of the Health Physics Society, Las Vegas, Nevada 1982.

27. Cliff KD, O'Riordan MC: Natural radioactivity in the countries of the European community. *Science Publ Policy* 1980; 281-288.

28. Harley J: Reports of Selected NCRP Activities. Eighteenth Annual Meeting of the National Council on Radiation Protection and Measurements, Washington DC, NCRP, 1982.

22.

Case Analysis: Health Hazards of Plutonium Release from the Rocky Flats Plant

Jeffrey V. Sutherland

The Rocky Flats Plant

The Rocky Flats Plant (RFP) is a key facility for production of nuclear weapons components for the U.S. Department of Defense. The plant fabricates plutonium "triggers" for new weapons and reprocesses plutonium from old weapons. Assembly of nuclear weapons components is accomplished at the Pantex Plant in Amarillo, Texas using plutonium components manufactured at Rocky Flats; electrical, mechanical, and explosive components are manufactured elsewhere in the country.[1] In addition to plutonium, the plant handles uranium, beryllium, and nitrate compounds, all of which are potential environmental hazards.

Plant construction at Rocky Flats started in 1951, and Dow Chemical Company began routine operations under an Atomic Energy Commission (AEC) contract in 1953.[2,3] Since 1953, the plant has experienced two major fires, a large release of plutonium-contaminated oil from rusting drums, and a release of radioactive tritium into the water supply of Broomfield, Colorado. The fires in 1957 and 1969 released an estimated 0.026 and 0.00086 curies, respectively, of plutonium into the offsite environment.[1] The 1957 actual release may have been several orders of magnitude higher than this estimate because no records of emissions were available during the fire and for seven days thereafter. Most of the present offsite contamination was caused by plutonium contaminated oil leaking from rusting barrels onto soil in an open storage area. The soil was blown outside plant boundaries, primarily during the period 1966-1969.[4] Krey[5] has estimated that a total of 3.4 ± 0.9 curies of Pu239 and Pu240 from Rocky Flats sources have been deposited on public and private lands. In 1973, an estimated 500–2000 curies of tritium were released into streams flowing off the Rocky Flats site as a result of processing plutonium with unexpected tritium contamination.[6]

213

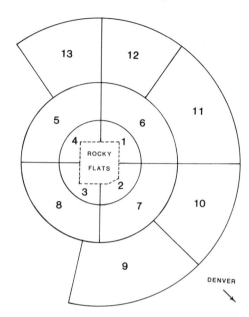

Figure 1. Sectors sampled by the Colorado Department of Health in the vicinity of the Rocky Flats Plant.

Levels of Soil Contamination Near The Rocky Flats Plant

A number of different soil-sampling techniques have been used in the RFP area, each producing different results. The major difference between techniques is the depth of soil sampled, although confusion is also caused by use of different units to describe contamination levels. The technique described by Krey[5] is considered most appropriate for determining total amounts of plutonium released by the plant. By sampling to a depth of 10 cm, this technique is able to measure about 90% of the total Rocky Flats plutonium deposition. For evaluation of health hazards, the Colorado Department of Health (CDH) uses a technique that samples the top 0.3 cm of soil. An alternative technique has been proposed by Johnson et al.[7] CDH[8] compared the latter two techniques and found that they yielded similar results. Average activity in the 13 sectors sampled by CDH (see Figure 1) was 6.28 disintegrations per minute per gram of dry soil (dpm/g) using the Johnson technique and 5.88 dpm/g using the CDH procedure. Spot variations were evident, particularly in sectors containing sharp concentration gradients.

Results of sampling for plutonium in contaminated soil in the vicinity of the RFP for the period 1970-1977 are presented in Table 1. The highest contamination is evident in areas south and southeast of the plant towards Denver. Contamination peaked in 1971 in Sector 2 at levels that were several hundred times those found in remote areas because of worldwide plutonium fallout. Isopleths indicating total plutonium deposition in soil from the data of

TABLE 1. ROCKY FLATS PLANT SURVEILLANCE. PLUTONIUM-239 CONCENTRATIONS IN SOIL (DPM/GM).

Immediate Vicinty Sector	1977	1976	1975	1974	1973	1972	1971	1970
1	2.28	1.51	—[a]	3.18	—	2.66	3.15	5.55
2	9.37	7.77	9.44	28.19	—	55.75	66.84	24.40
3	0.22	0.36	0.49	0.36	—	0.17	0.07	0.29
4	0.20	0.27	0.22	0.45	—	0.22	0.29	0.31
5	0.13	0.08	0.13	0.70	—	0.33	0.37	0.24
6	0.66	0.24	<0.02	0.48	0.15	0.71	0.63	1.00
7	0.64	0.27	0.29	0.80	0.83	0.57	0.79	1.02
8	0.16	0.13	0.16	0.29	—	0.24	0.60	0.04
9	0.13	0.16	0.09	0.04	0.07	0.31	0.29	0.02
10	0.22	0.16	—	0.17	0.11	0.20	0.12	0.38
11	0.07	0.04	—	0.23	0.14	0.18	0.12	0.07
12	0.06	0.07	0.07	0.19	—	0.15	0.06	0.02
13	0.07	0.09	0.07	0.13	—	<0.04	0.12	0.04
Remote Sites								
Loveland	0.02	—	—	—	0.12	—	0.10	0.11
Livermore	<0.02	0.02	—	—	0.04	0.07	<0.04	0.04
Crooke	0.04	0.08	—	—	0.05	0.11	0.13	0.04
Burlington	0.07	0.02	—	—	0.05	0.07	0.11	0.09
Limon	0.04	0.04	—	—	0.06	0.07	0.06	0.13
Springfield	0.02	0.02	0.04	—	<0.04	0.12	0.09	0.04
Walsenburg	0.04	—	0.02	—	0.05	0.11	0.07	0.11
Penrose	0.04	0.09	—	—	0.06	0.11	0.08	0.11

[a]—Indicates that no analysis results were available on this sample. *(From CDH 1977, p. 18.)*

Krey and Hardy[9] are presented in Figure 2. Units in this figure are millicuries of plutonium per square kilometer (mCi/km²). Total deposition in mCi/km² in the Krey and Hardy data is consistent with values for surface deposition in dpm/g in the CDH[8] data.

Plutonium Toxicology

General biomedical aspects of plutonium exposure are discussed at length by Hodge et al.[10] Because of the lack of human data on the effects of plutonium exposure, risk estimates have been based on the results of animal experiments and on the extrapolation of data for radium dial painters.[11-13]

The route of exposure from soil contamination in the RFP area is primarily through inhalation. Bair et al.[14] reviewed data on inhalation exposure and noted that 70 nCi of plutonium deposited in a beagle's lungs is sufficient to cause cancer in 100% of the dogs living more than 1600 days (no neoplasia was evident in controls). The maximum permission body burden (MPBB) for a plutonium worker is 40 nCi. However, the maximum permissible lung bur-

ROCKY FLATS

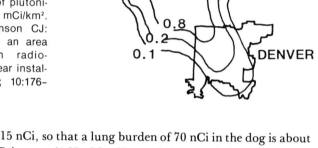

Figure 2. Isopleths of plutonium soil deposition in mCi/km². (Redrawn from Johnson CJ: Cancer incidence in an area contaminated with radionuclides near a nuclear installation. Ambio, 1981; 10:176–182.)

den (MPLB) is only 15 nCi, so that a lung burden of 70 nCi in the dog is about five times the MPLB in man.[14] Health effects of alpha-emitting particles in the respiratory tract have been reviewed by the British Medical Research Council,[15] NCRP,[16] The BEIR Committee,[17] and Bair and Thomas.[18]

Movement of plutonium out of the lung into other organs is affected by the type of isotope and/or chemical compound present. Alveolar-deposited Pu239 dioxide has been studied in the dog.[19] The half-life of this plutonium compound in the lung is about 800 days. It moves from the lung primarily into the thoracic lymph nodes. A substantial amount (about 25% after 3 years) eventually settles in the liver, skeleton, and abdominal lymph nodes. Smaller amounts settle in the gonads in animals and humans.[20]

Previously Developed Risk Estimates

Risk estimates of the hazards of plutonium soil contamination in the vicinity of Rocky Flats have been developed by the Department of Energy (DOE), the Environmental Protection Agency (EPA), and CDH. For persons living in areas with soil contamination levels of 20 mCi/km² (100 times background), the EPA[21] risk model estimates 0.018 cancer deaths per year per million people exposed. A DOE[22] Environmental Dispersion Model estimates the risk to be 0.03 deaths per million person-years exposure at this level. CDH[23] assessed the risk of living in an area with soil contaminated to a level of the Colorado state standard (2 dpm/g which is equivalent to 3.34 mCi/km²). Multiplying the CDH risk estimate by 20/3.34 yields 0.216 estimated cancer deaths per million person-years at risk. This is an order of magnitude higher than Federal estimates.

It must be emphasized that such estimates are sensitive to parameter values specified in the various mathematical models used to generate them. The mathematical models are not readily available in the scientific literature and are not easily understood even by an expert in the field. All estimates quoted above rely on the BEIR I[24] Committee report on the effects of ionizing radiation. The publication of the BEIR III[25] report in 1980 provided new information for use in risk estimation.

THE ROCKY FLATS MONITORING COMMITTEE

The Rocky Flats Monitoring Committee (RFMC), established in Colorado by Governor Richard Lamm and Congressman Tim Wirth, has been given the responsibility for monitoring the RFP. A Governor's Executive Order of June 8, 1978, included the following mandate:

> to provide state and local government officials with continuous advice (regarding) . . . the welfare of local citizens; to conduct an extensive information program to educate the public about the Rocky Flats Plant; to study and evaluate reports, accidents and various health standards applicable to the Rocky Flats Plant and to educate the public about the same.

After reviewing the data summarized previously, the Monitoring Committee concluded that available evidence was insufficient to advise the public concerning inconsistencies in estimates of risk, and that monitoring cancer rates in the vicinity of the RFP was essential to provide assurance to the public that no excess risk was present, or that a specific level of hazard was to be expected by residents living in the area. For this purpose the RFMC requested that the Colorado legislature substantially increase its funding of the CDH Central Cancer Registry.

Concurrently, the RFMC requested that the University of Colorado School of Medicine (UCSM) review epidemiologic studies related to the assessment of risk of plutonium inhalation and to initiate new studies, as appropriate, for refining estimates of hazards associated with working at or living near the RFP.

REVIEW OF EPIDEMIOLOGIC STUDIES OF RISK OF PLUTONIUM EXPOSURE

Studies of Morbidity in Populations Near Nuclear Facilities

Adequate epidemiological data on human cancer incidence is unavailable for populations not occupationally exposed to internal deposition of alpha-emitting radionuclides. Tokuhata and Smith[26] reviewed health studies of populations living near nuclear facilities and found a single morbidity study in the literature. Moshman and Holland[27] reported cancer incidence for Oak Ridge was 123 per 100,000 person-years at risk compared to a national average of 230 per 100,000. This rate was age-adjusted to 13 different state standard populations where cancer incidence data was available for comparison. Results were too variable for conclusions to be drawn. Although respiratory cancers in males were higher than expected, this was explained as possibly due to generally rising lung cancer rates. It should be noted that the Oak Ridge population of approximately 300,000 had an average length of residence of 9.8 months. Since the latent period of even the most rapidly appearing cancers is significantly longer than 9.8 months, any radiation-induced cancers appearing in this population would probably be due to exposures received elsewhere.

More recently, Voelz and Stebbings[28] have reported cancer incidence in Los Alamos County, New Mexico, for the period 1969-1974. The age-adjusted rate for all malignant neoplasms was 420.2 per 100,000 versus 311.0 per 100,000 for the entire New Mexico population. Rates of cancers of the pancreas, bladder, and digestive system were elevated, whereas cancers of the respiratory system and leukemias and lymphomas were about the same as the New Mexico population. Small numbers (62 total cancers) preclude drawing definitive conclusions. It should be noted that most Los Alamos families have someone employed at the Los Alamos National Laboratory.

Berg and Finch[29] analyzed cancer incidence rates in the area of Rocky Flats at the request of Dr. Carl Johnson, former Director of the Jefferson County Health Department. Johnson[30] reported elevated observed/expected ratios near Rocky Flats for male lung, and male and female colon and rectal cancers. Overall cancer rates in a population of 154,170 people living closest to the plant were 24% higher in male and 10% higher in females than rates in 423,870 persons living in a control area at a distance from the plant. A downward gradient in excess cancers was noted for both males and females in groups located in four areas with plutonium soil contamination of 48-0.8 mCi/km^2, 0.8-0.2 mCi/km^2, 0.2-0.1 mCi/km^2, and less than 0.1 mCi/km^2 respectively.

An unpublished analysis of these data by UCSM epidemiologists has shown that adjusting the cancer rates for socioeconomic status indicates that the elevated rates are specific to lower socioeconomic groups. Adjustment for other confounding factors such as smoking, mobility, other exposures, etc., has not been accomplished.

Even if these estimates were valid after adjustment for possible confounding factors, the causal relationship between plutonium exposure and neoplastic transformation remains tenuous. Poet and Martel[4] reported that most of the plutonium soil contamination in the Rocky Flats area occurred during the period 1966-1969. It is highly unlikely that this source of exposure could induce excess cancer during 1969-1971. The fire which occurred in 1957 could have resulted in substantial doses of plutonium to the lungs of persons living downwind from the plant at that time. However, most of the release was not measured due to a power outage at the Plant, so dose estimates remain speculative.

Chinn[31] reanalyzed the Third National Cancer Survey Colorado data and obtained results similar to those of Johnson. After controlling for race, age, sex, income, and air pollution, cancer risk in the most contaminated area was 10% higher than in the Denver Standard Metropolitan Statistical Area which includes Denver, Boulder, Jefferson, Araphoe, and Douglas counties. Out of 125 excess cancer cases, 90 were in organs considered radiosensitive by the ICRP. Chinn did not remove Spanish surnamed persons from the data prior to analysis as in the Berg/Johnson data. This could distort the findings if few people of Spanish surname live near the plant, since such people have much lower cancer rates than other Caucasians.

Studies of Mortality in Populations Near Nuclear Facilities

Mortality studies are inherently less precise and powerful than incidence studies. While cancers of the lung, pancreas, and some leukemias produce less than 10% five-year relative survival rates, thyroid cancers have an 84% ten-year relative survival rate in whites.[32] High survival rates mean that mortality is far removed in time from the initial exposure to carcinogenic agents and also imply reduced power due to smaller sample sizes for a mortality versus incidence study on the same population. In addition, case ascertainment using death certificates is variable for different neoplasms and for different times and places. Jablon et al.[33] completed a population death certificate study in Japan and discovered only 75% of cancer deaths are identified on death certificates. The identification rate for leukemia was quite high at 92%, but this was in Hiroshima and Nagasaki where researchers were looking for radiation effects. It is not surprising, therefore, that low-dose radiation studies of cancer mortality in human populations have produced conflicting, and often negative, results.

Studies on health effects of uranium mill tailings are a case in point. Although Mason and coworkers[34] found no increase in 1950–1969 cancer mortality attributable to uranium mill tailings in Colorado, the CDH[35] identified an increase in lung cancer and leukemia incidence in Mesa County (including the city of Grand Junction, where extensive tailings deposits exist) for the period 1970–1976. A follow-up mortality study based on interviews of relatives of deceased leukemia patients was undertaken by the CDH to determine if cases were occurring in persons living in residences built on discarded mill tailings. The study produced negative results but utilized mortality experience during the period evaluated by Mason and coworkers. Perhaps the period between deposition of mill tailings (late 1950s, early 1960s) and the midpoint of the mortality study (1968) was shorter than the latency period for induction of leukemia from very low exposure to radiation.

The elevated lung and leukemia incidence rates during the period 1970–1976 remain unexplained. However, work in this area is of continuing interest.[36] Exposure to radon gas from uranium mill tailings results in a low-level exposure to internal alpha-emitting particles. This is the only low-level radiation exposure to a large population which is similar to inhalation of plutonium particles resuspended from contaminated soil.

Takuhata and Smith[26] reviewed mortality studies of populations not occupationally exposed living near nuclear facilities and noted no clearly positive results. Bailar and Young[37] studied cancer mortality rates in counties downstream from the Hanford nuclear facility in the state of Washington. No excess risk of death from cancer was noted. Several investigators[38-43] have investigated infant mortality and other indices of radiation health effects on populations living near nuclear facilities. Only Sternglass[40] has claimed consistent positive correlations between infant mortality and low-level radiation releases from nuclear reactors. His experimental design and method of adjustment of rates for possible confounding factors have generated unresolved questions about his conclusions.

Studies of Occupationally Exposed Populations

Studies of radiation effects on occupationally exposed personnel working in nuclear facilities have generally produced inconclusive results due to small sample sizes and the lack of appropriate controls. Radiation workers are healthier than unselected populations and usually have lower cancer rates than the U.S. population (the healthy worker effect). Larson et al.[44] examined worker death rates at the Oak Ridge nuclear facility for the period 1950-1965. Only 692 deaths occurred, compared to 992 expected based on U.S. mortality rates. This difference was attributed to the healthy worker effect. Scott et al.[45] compared deaths in uranium workers versus deaths in nonuranium workers for the period 1951-1969 and found uranium workers had 59% higher mortality than that expected on the basis of 1960 U.S. mortality rates in the general population. However, non-uranium workers had mortality 76% higher than the U.S. population. These findings are likely to be due to bias in the selection of case and control groups.

Voelz et al.[46] have followed up 26 Manhattan Project plutonium workers and found no unusual morbidity or mortality effects. However, these findings suggest only that there are no gross effects from levels of 6-230 nCi of plutonium systemic body burden. For example, no lung cancers have been found in this group, but only 0.25 lung cancers would be expected on the basis of U.S. general population rates. A mortality study of 224 Los Alamos workers with plutonium burdens greater than or equal to 10 nCi has also been completed[28] with negative results. However, these workers have been highly selected for security clearances and specialized work. The healthy worker effect should produce lower cancer rates than U.S. national averages. In addition, only seven neoplasms were found among these workers. If a proper control group had been selected and seven cases observed in the control group, this experimental design would have a 90% chance of detecting a relative risk of 8.0 if such a risk existed. In order to have a 90% chance of detecting a 10% increase in risk, 3,776 cases of cancer would need to be observed in the study population.[47] Clearly, this study is inadequate to rule out a small increase in the risk of cancer in Los Alamos workers.

Chromosome breakage dose-response effects in RFP plutonium workers have been reported by Brandom et al.[48] Effects were similar to those discovered in nuclear dockyard workers.[49] The relationship between chromosome breakage and other health effects is uncertain. However, Kochupillai et al.[50] found cytogenetic aberrations in people living in Kerala, India, where background levels of radiation are 1500–3000 mrem per year. Prevalence of severe mental retardation of genetic origin was four times higher in the study population than in a control population living in villages with 100 mrem per year background levels of radiation. This suggests the possibility of health effects of low-level plutonium exposure in offspring of plutonium workers.

Voelz et al.[51] analyzed mortality in 7112 white males who worked at the RFP during the period 1952–1979. No significant increase in cancer rates was observed compared to U.S. population rates (another example of the healthy worker effect). This study failed to compare adequately the exposed versus nonexposed workers. In addition, the mean age of the cohort was 48 years — too young to observe the appearance of many cancers. This study, therefore, remains inconclusive.

Mancuso et al.[52] reported an increased risk of certain malignant neoplasms for Hanford employees exposed to external radiation. Original data have been extended and reanalyzed.[53] Results have been extensively debated in the literature.[54-60] Marks et al.[57] and Reissland[59] concur with the Mancuso finding of excess cancer of the pancreas and multiple myeloma in Hanford workers. There appears, however, to be a deficit of leukemias in this worker population, suggesting lack of exposure to excess external radiation. Lung cancer rates may be high for Hanford workers,[55] but the data have not been adjusted for possible confounding factors, particularly smoking. If lung cancer rates remained elevated after accounting for possible confounding factors, internal exposure to alpha-emitting nuclides would be an alternative hypothesis for explaining the data. A possible relationship between alpha-emitting radionuclides and pancreatic cancer has previously been observed in Mesa County, Colorado,[61] an area with elevated levels of radon gas emitted from abandoned uranium mill tailings.

The effect of radon exposure on uranium miners has been well documented.[62-70] Lundin[66] reported excess lung cancer in 3,366 white and 780 nonwhite uranium miners exposed to radon daughter levels of more than 120 working-level-months (about 20 rem). Archer et al.[71] showed that the uranium miner data from the United States, Canada, and several European countries suggest that the linear hypothesis may underestimate the effects of low-level radiation exposure for internally deposited alpha-emitting radionuclides. Radford[72] reviewed data on miners exposed to radon daughters and noted that Czechoslovakian, Newfoundland, and Swedish miners have 3–5 times the increase in risk of cancer as U.S. uranium miners. He concluded that either U.S. uranium miner dose estimates are inflated, or that very high doses produce less effect per rad than small doses.

DEVELOPING ESTIMATES OF RISK FOR PERSONS LIVING NEAR THE RFP

Review of the literature shows that few studies are directly applicable to estimating the risk of living near the Rocky Flats Plant. Studies of plutonium workers have produced negative findings, but do not have the ability to detect small increases in risk because of the small study populations, inadequate analyses, or youthful cohorts. Cancer incidence during 1969–1971 appeared slightly elevated near the RFP compared to control areas. However, controversy exists as to the cause of these increased rates.

Education of the public concerning the health risk of RFP operations was impaired by disagreements among scientific experts as to risk of exposure to plutonium in the environment. As a result, the RFMC asked the University of Colorado Center for Research on Judgment and Policy (CRJP) for assistance in February, 1981.

It became apparent that the most productive means of clarifying the controversy surrounding the RFP was to "externalize" the process of expert judgment, that is, to identify the data, assumptions, and analytic principles used by experts to evaluate risk of plutonium exposure. The CRJP showed that it would be possible to move the discussion of risk from the arena of intuitive judgment (often with data unknown) to aided judgment (where data, assumptions, and analytic principles are clearly specified). A three-phase study directed towards externalization of the judgment process was initiated.

Phase I

In Phase I of the study, Hammond and Marvin[73] documented the sources of disagreement among 11 scientists who were asked to judge risk of plutonium exposure for individuals with various confounding factors. Five of the scientists were epidemiologists, four were biostatisticians, and two were medical physicists.

The intuitive judgments developed by the scientists were shown to be based on stable self-consistent judgement policies. However, risk estimates were highly variable. The sources of disagreement were not directly associated with professional background and training but were based on the characteristics of the individual judgement policies. The principles on which the scientists organized information appeared to be a more important factor in generating differences than the relative weights given by each scientist to confounding variables influencing risk of plutonium exposure.

Phase II

Results from Phase I of this study indicated that "externalization" of the judgment process might bring about better agreement among scientists as to the health risk of the RFP. Five of the most widely disagreeing scientists from Phase I (including all cancer epidemiologists in the Denver area) were asked to participate in Phase II. They were individually interviewed and asked (1) "What is the best available data published in the scientific literature which is relevant to health risks of plutonium exposure from the RFP?" and (2) "What are the most appropriate, clearly defined, analytical principles with which to evaluate this data?" At the end of several interview cycles all five scientists independently concluded that lung cancer was the primary risk from plutonium released from the RFP to the environment and agreed on basic principles for estimating the risk of exposure to airborne plutonium.[74] These principles have been followed in the development of the risk estimation procedure discussed below.

The process of obtaining judgments was not one of developing a consensus. Efforts were made to avoid development of group opinion. Only individuals were interviewed. The only information that passed from one expert to another was a specific reference to the literature or a proposed analytic principle based on a reference in the literature.

Expert judgment was considered irrelevant without appropriate data in the literature to substantiate that judgment, with one exception. Insufficient data is available in the literature to support or refute the hypothesis that the dose-response curve for exposure to radon daughters has the same shape as the dose-response curve for persons exposed to plutonium aerosols.

Phase III

In Phase III of this study, a panel of four experts in health physics developed an analytical procedure for estimation of dose to the lung from airborne plutonium. This procedure was used in combination with principles developed in Phase II to estimate risk of exposure.

Risk Estimation Procedures

Estimation of the relative risk of lung cancer for an individual with specific age, smoking status, and plutonium exposure, compared to a nonsmoking individual of the same age exposed only to worldwide plutonium fallout, was accomplished as follows:

1. Individual age, average number of cigarettes smoked per day, average ambient air level of Pu239 + 240 in microcuries per cubic

meter of air, and time of exposure to this ambient air level were specified.

2. The cumulative dose in rem to the lung from chronic low-level exposure to plutonium from the RFP was calculated.

3. The expected incidence of lung cancer for persons of the same age and smoking status was calculated using the equation of Doll and Peto[75] for smokers, and the data of Doll and Hill,[76] Hammond[77] and Kahn[78] for nonsmokers.

4. The expected incidence of lung cancer for persons of the same age and smoking status was adjusted for working level months equivalent radon exposure using the data of Archer et al.[79]

5. The relative risk of lung cancer was estimated by dividing the incidence rate calculated in (4) by the expected incidence of lung cancer in nonsmokers with no Rocky Flats plutonium exposure.

The equation developed for determining the incidence of lung cancer per 100,000 per year in persons of age A, who began smoking C cigarettes per day between ages 16-25 was:

$$I = (0.273 \times 10^{-7}) (C + 6)^2 (A - 22.5)^{4.5} \exp [0.00018 (\text{Dose})].$$

The first part of the equation represents risk from smoking alone.[75] The last part, $\exp [0.00018 (\text{Dose})]$, represents the increased risk from plutonium exposure and the interaction effect between cigarette smoking and plutonium inhalation.

Development of procedures for estimation of dose and the risk equation above is discussed in detail by Sutherland.[80] Here, it should be noted that the BEIR III Committee[25] concluded that available data suggest that alpha irradiation/smoking risk could be most accurately estimated by a function which included both additive and multiplicative components. The equation above is approximately linear in the low-dose region for fixed age and smoking status, indicating that risk of plutonium exposure is additive. In the high-dose region, there is both an additive and multiplicative effect.

Calculation of Relative Risk of Lung Cancer

Calculation of relative risk is accomplished by dividing the estimated incidence of lung cancer for persons with specified age, smoking status, and plutonium exposure by the expected incidence of lung cancer in nonsmokers with no Rocky Flats plutonium exposure. Eight ambient air levels of Rocky Flats Pu239 + 240 were chosen for analysis (see Table 2) based on the data of Barker[81] concerning levels of ambient air plutonium at the east gate of the plant during 1974-1978 (see Figure 3). The first level presented [level (0)] was for no Rocky Flats plutonium exposure. Relative risks in Tables 3 and 4 for

TABLE 2. AMBIENT AIR LEVELS OF PU239 + 240

Description	Level	μCi/m³
No exposure	0	0.0
Typical background fallout	1	0.1×10^{-9}
Low RFP sampler east gate	2	0.5×10^{-9}
Typical RFP sample east gate	3	0.1×10^{-8}
Typical EML sample east gate	4	0.2×10^{-8}
Typical CDH sample east gate	5	0.5×10^{-8}
DOE/CDH guideline	6	0.6×10^{-7}
Less than 1/50 of 1957 release	7	0.1×10^{-5}

this level reflect age and smoking risk only. Level (1), 0.1×10^{-9} μCi of Pu239 + 240/m³ of air, is a typical background level recorded at CDH in metropolitan Denver. No increase in risk is noted at background fallout levels.

Risk of Living Near the RFP During 1974–1978

Level (2), 0.5×10^{-9} μCi/m³, was the *lowest* average reading reported from RFP east gate samples during the years 1974–1978. Levels (3), (4), and (5) are *typical* levels reported from RFP, DOE Environmental Measurements Laboratory (EML), and CDH samplers respectively during the same period $(0.1 \times 10^{-8}, 0.2 \times 10^{-8}, 0.5 \times 10^{-8} \mu$Ci/m³).

No increase in radiation risk is noticeable at these levels of plutonium exposure in any age group at any smoking level. Under normal operating conditions during 1974–1978, the plant presented no noticeable radiation hazard to persons living in its vicinity [compare levels (2), (3), and (4) in Tables 3 and 4].

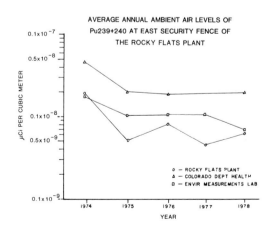

Figure 3. Average annual ambient air levels of Pu239 + 240 at the east security fence of the Rocky Flats Plant during 1974–1978 as measured by three different agencies.

TABLE 3. LUNG CANCER RELATIVE RISK FOR NONSMOKING WHITE MALES

Age	Plutonium ambient air levels							
	(0)	(1)	(2)	(3)	(4)	(5)	(6)	(7)
40	1.00	1.00	1.00	1.00	1.00	1.00	1.00	1.06
45	1.00	1.00	1.00	1.00	1.00	1.00	1.00	1.06
50	1.00	1.00	1.00	1.00	1.00	1.00	1.00	1.07
55	1.00	1.00	1.00	1.00	1.00	1.00	1.00	1.08
60	1.00	1.00	1.00	1.00	1.00	1.00	1.01	1.09
65	1.00	1.00	1.00	1.00	1.00	1.00	1.01	1.10
70	1.00	1.00	1.00	1.00	1.00	1.00	1.01	1.10
75	1.00	1.00	1.00	1.00	1.00	1.00	1.01	1.11

Risk of Plutonium Exposure at DOE/CDH Guidelines

Level (6), 0.6×10^{-7} υCi/m^3, is the DOE/CDH guideline for release of soluble plutonium aerosols in controlled areas. At this level of exposure, a 1% increase in relative risk is noted for nonsmokers. A similar percentage increase is noted for smokers. Since no noticeable increase in risk should be observable at DOE/CDH guideline exposures, this guideline needs more careful evaluation by federal and state regulatory authorities.

Risk of Plutonium Exposure Under Accident Conditions

During 1957, a fire and explosion at the plant produced unmonitored plutonium releases during the fire and for six days thereafter due to power outage. Monitoring resumed seven days after the fire and recorded a release equal to 50 years exposure at level (7). Actual release may have been an order of magnitude or more greater.[30]

Therefore, some individuals downwind from the plant may have received

TABLE 4. LUNG CANCER RELATIVE RISK FOR WHITE MALE SMOKERS (20 CIGARETTES PER DAY)

Age	Plutonium ambient air levels							
	(0)	(1)	(2)	(3)	(4)	(5)	(6)	(7)
40	2.82	2.82	2.82	2.82	2.82	2.82	2.83	2.98
45	5.34	5.34	5.34	5.34	5.35	5.35	5.36	5.69
50	8.50	8.50	8.50	8.50	8.50	8.50	8.53	9.11
55	12.11	12.11	12.11	12.11	12.11	12.12	12.17	13.08
60	16.04	16.04	16.04	16.04	16.05	16.05	16.12	17.46
65	20.18	20.18	20.18	20.18	20.18	20.19	20.29	22.12
70	24.44	24.44	24.44	24.44	24.45	24.45	24.59	26.99
75	28.76	28.76	28.76	28.76	28.76	28.77	28.94	31.99

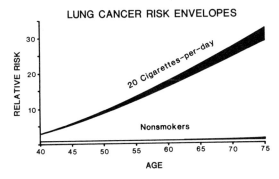

LUNG CANCER RISK ENVELOPES

Figure 4. Lung cancer risk envelopes for white males—20 cigarettes per day versus no smoking ages. The lower bound is for background levels of plutonium exposure, while the upper bound is for exposure at level (7) which has been exceeded only under accident conditions.

a cumulative dose in 1957 equivalent to more than 50 years exposure at level (7). The increase in risk for lifetime exposure at level (7) (see Tables 3 and 4) varies from 4% for 40 year old males to 11% for 75 year old males. It is essential, therefore, that the Rocky Flats Emergency Response Plan allow for evacuation of persons living near the plant in the event of an accident.

Relationship Between Plutonium Risk and Smoking Habits
While radiation risk percentage increases are similar for smokers and non-smokers, smoking alone increases the risk of lung cancer much more than possible increases in risk from past Rocky Flats Plant operations. For non-smokers, the relative risk of lung cancer varies from 1.0 at level (5) to 1.11 at level (7). For persons smoking 20 cigarettes/day, relative risk increased from 28.77 at level (5) to 31.99 at level (7). In both cases, for a 75 year old male, the increase was 11% over this range of plutonium exposures.

Risk envelopes are plotted in Figure 4 for white males at different ages and smoking levels. The lower bound of the envelopes is the risk of lung cancer without any plutonium exposure (except for worldwide fallout levels). The upper bound is the risk at level (7) which has been exceeded only under accident conditions.

Potential sources of error in these risk estimates are discussed by Sutherland.[80] Radiation scientists have questioned the validity of using radon exposures to estimate risk of plutonium exposure, although it is generally agreed that no other data exist that are more relevant. Also, recent data on miners exposed to radon at lower levels than U.S. uranium miners suggest that risk may be higher per unit dose by a factor of two.[82]

CONCLUSION

In summary, no increase in risk was noted for ambient air levels of Pu239 + 240 measured at the east gate of the Rocky Flats Plant during 1974-1978. An 11% increase in risk for 75 year old smokers and nonsmokers was estimated for lifetime exposure to 0.1×10^{-5} μCi/m³ of air. This level was exceeded onsite by a factor of 50 in 1957 due to an accident at the plant. Citizens living downwind from the plant, particularly during the 1957 fire, could be placed at a small increased relative risk (see Tables 3 and 4 and Figure 4).

While the percentage increase in risk for smokers and nonsmokers is identical for various exposure levels, the additional estimated numbers of lung cancer cases induced will occur primarily in smokers since smoking appears to be a far greater hazard than levels of plutonium exposure evaluated. Increased involuntary risks from plutonium exposure may occur primarily as the result of risks undertaken voluntarily by those who smoke cigarettes.

REFERENCES

1. LWTF: Lamm-Wirth Task Force on Rocky Flats, Final Report, 1975. State of Colorado (Office of the Governor).
2. AEC: Environmental Statement: Land Acquisition, Rocky Flats Plant, Colorado. U.S. Atomic Energy Commission WASH-1518, 1972, Washington, DC.
3. AEC: Environmental Statement: Plutonium Recovery Facility, Rocky Flats Plant, Colorado. U.S. Atomic Energy Commission WASH-1507, 1972, Washington, DC.
4. Poet SE, Martell EA: Plutonium-239 and americium-241 contamination in the Denver area. *Health Phys* 1972; 23:537-548.
5. Krey PW: Remote plutonium contamination and total inventories from Rocky Flats. *Health Phys* 1976; 30:209-214.
6. EPA: Investigative Report of the 1973 Tritium Release at the Rocky Flats Plant in Golden, Colorado. Radiation/Noise Control Branch, Hazardous Materials Control Division, US Environmental Protection Agency, 1975, Washington DC.
7. Johnson CJ, Tidball RR, Severson RC: Plutonium hazard in respirable dust on the surface of soil. *Science* 1976; 193:488-490.
8. CDH: Radioactive soil contamination (cesium-137 and plutonium) in the environment near the Rocky Flats Nuclear Weapons Plant. Colorado Department of Health, Denver, 1977.
9. Krey PW, Hardy EP: Plutonium in Soil Around the Rocky Flats Plant. Health Safety Laboratory, U.S. Atomic Energy Commission HASL-235, 1970, New York.
10. Hodge HC, Stannard JN, Hursh JB (Eds): *Handbook of Experimental Pharmacology*, Vol. XXXVI New York: Springer-Verlag, 1973.
11. Rowland RE, Stehney AF, Lucas HF Jr: Dose-response relationships for female radium dial workers. *Rad Res* 1978; 76:368-383.
12. Marshall JH, Groer PG, Schlenker RA: Dose to endosteal cells and relative distribution factors for radium-224 and plutonium-329 compared to radium-226. *Health Phys* 1978; 35:91-101.
13. Rowland RE: The risk of bone sarcoma from plutonium-239. *International*

Symposium on Biological Implications of Radionuclides Released from Nuclear Industries IAEA-SM-237/55, Vienna, March, 1979. pp. 26-30.

14. Bair WJ, Ballou JE, Park JF, et al.: Plutonium in soft tissues with emphasis on the respiratory tract. In: *Handbook of Experimental Pharmacology* Vol. XXXVI (HC Hodge, JN Stannard, JB Hursh, Eds.) New York: Springer-Verlag, 1973. pp 503-568.

15. Medical Research Council: *The Toxicity of Plutonium*. Her Majesty's Stationery Office, London 1975. pp 1-38.

16. NCRP: Alpha-emitting particles in lungs: Recommendations of the NCRP. Natl Council on Radiat Protection Measurements Rep 46, 1975, Washington DC.

17. BEIR: Report of Ad Hoc Committee on "Hot Particles": Health Effects of Alpha-Emitting Particles in the Respiratory Tract. Advisory Committee on Biological Effects Ionizing Radiat, Natl Academy Sciences, 1976, Washington DC.

18. Bair WJ, Thomas JM: Prediction of the health effects of inhaled transuranium elements from experimental animal data. *Proc IAEA Symp* Vienna, IAEA-SM-199/58.

19. Park JF, Bair WJ, Busch RH: Progress in beagle dog studies with transuranium elements at Batelle-Northwest. *Health Phys* 1972; 22:803-810.

20. Russell JJ, Lindenbaum A: One-year study of nonuniformly distributed plutonium in mouse testis as related to spermatogonial irradiation. Health Phys 1979; 36:153-157.

21. EPA: Persons exposed to transuranium elements in the environment: Federal radiation protection guidance on dose limits. Environment Protection Agency, Federal Register, November 30, 1977. pp 60956-60959.

22. DOE: Defendant's analysis of health risks of the contaminated lands. Department Energy Pretrial Statement Exhibit D. Marcus Church, Good Realty, Great Western Venture vs ERDA, Dow Chemical Co, Rockwell International Corp.

23. CDH: A risk evaluation for the Colorado plutonium-in-soil standard. Colorado Department of Health, 1976.

24. BEIR: The Effects on Populations of Exposure to Low Levels of Ionizing Radiation. Advisory Committee on Biological Effects of Ionizing Radiation, Natl Academy Sciences, 1972, Washington DC.

25. BEIR: The Effects on Populations of Exposure to Low Levels of Ionizing Radiation: 1980. Washington: National Academy Press, 1980.

26. Tokuhata GK: Smith MW, History of health studies related to nuclear facilities: A methodological consideration. Second Workshop on Health Surveillance Around Point Sources of Pollution, Albuquerque, January 22-24, 1979.

27. Moshman MA, Holland AH: On the incidence of cancer in Oak Ridge, Tennessee. *Cancer* 1949; 2:567-575.

28. Voelz GL, Stebbings JH, Hempelmann LH, et al.: Studies on persons exposed to plutonium. Int Atomic Energy Agency Symposium on Late Biological Effects Ionizing Radiat IAEA-SM-224/508, Vienna, March 13-17, 1978. pp 353-367.

29. Berg JW, Finch J: Unpublished data. Colorado Regional Cancer Center Inc, Denver.

30. Johnson CJ: Cancer incidence in an area contaminated with radionuclides near a nuclear installation. *Ambio* 1981; 10:176-182.

31. Chinn S: The relation of the Rocky Flats plant and other factors to 1969-71

cancer incidence in the Denver area. Denver: Fairfield and Woods, 1981.

32.   Axtell LM, Ardyce JA, Myers MH: Cancer Patient Survival, Report Number 5. DHEW Pub No (NIH) 77-992, 1976.

33.   Jablon S, Angevine DM, Matsumoto YS, et al.: On the significance of cause of death as recorded on death certificates in Hiroshima and Nagasaki, *Jpn Natl Cancer Inst Monogr* 1965; 19:445-465.

34.   Mason TJ, Fraumeni JF, McKay FW: Uranium mill tailings and cancer mortality in Colorado. *J Natl Cancer Inst* 1972; 49:661-664.

35.   CDH: Leukemia in Mesa County: A follow-up. Colorado Department Health Weekly Dis Summary 36, 1979.

36.   Carter LJ: Uranium mill tailings: Congress addresses a long-neglected problem. *Science* 1978; 202:191-195.

37.   Bailar JC III, Young JL: Oregon malignancy pattern and radioisotope storage. *Pub Health Rep* 1966; 81:311-317.

38.   Tompkins EA, Hamilton PM, Hoffman DA: Infant mortality around three nuclear power reactors. In: *Proceedings of the Sixth Berkeley Symposium on Mathematical Statistics Probability* Vol IV. (LeCam LM, Neyman J, Eds) Berkeley: Univ California Press, 1972. pp 279-289.

39.   DeGroot MH: Statistical studies of the effect of low level radiation from nuclear reactors on human health. In: *Proceedings Sixth Berkeley Symposium on Mathematical Statistics Probability* Vol VI. (LeCam LM, Neyman J, Eds) Berkeley: Univ California Press, 1972. pp 223-234.

40.   Sternglass EJ: Environmental radiation and human health. In: *Proceedings of the Sixth Berkeley Symposium on Mathematical Statistics Probability* Vol IV. (LeCam LM, Neyman J, Eds) Berkeley: Univ California Press, 1972.

41.   Johnson MF, Foleman GR: The health effects of exposure to low-level radiation from nuclear power plants: A feasibility study. Presented at Health Phys Soc Meeting, New York, 1975.

42.   NYDH: Summary of Selected Health Statistics for Counties with Nuclear Facilities: New York State Excluding New York City, 1960-1975. New York Dept of Health, Monograph 13, Albany, NY, August, 1977.

43.   Patrick CH: Trends in public health in the population near nuclear facilities: A critical assessment. *Nuclear Safety* 1977; 18:647-662.

44.   Larson CE, Lincoln TA, Bahler KW: Comparison of Mortality of Union Carbide Employees in Oak Ridge Atomic Energy Facilities with U.S. Bureau Vital Statistics Mortality. U.S. Atomic Energy Commission Rep K-A-708, Oak Ridge Gaseous Diffusion Plant, NTIS, June 9, 1966.

45.   Scott LM, Bahler KW, De La Garza A, et al.: Mortality experience of uranium and nonuranium workers. *Health Phys* 1972; 23:555-557.

46.   Voelz GL, Hempelmann L, Lawrence JNP, et al.: A thirty-two year medical follow-up of Manhattan Project plutonium workers. *Health Phys*, 1979 37:445-485.

47.   Gail M: Power computations for designing comparative Poisson trials. *Biometrics* 1974; 30:231-237.

48.   Brandom WF, Archer PG, Bloom AD, et al.: Chromosome changes in somatic cells of workers with internal depositions of plutonium. In: *Biological Implications Radionuclides Released from Nuclear Industries* II, IAEA-SM-237/38, Vienna, 1979. pp 195-210.

49. Evans HJ, Buckton KE, Hamilton GE, et al.: Radiation-induced chromosome aberrations in nuclear-dockyard workers. *Nature* 1979; 277:531-534.

50. Kochupillai N, Verma IC, Grewal MS, et al.: Down's syndrome and related abnormalities in an area of high background radiation in coastal Kerala. *Nature* 1976; 262:60-61.

51. Voelz GL, Wilkinson GS, Acquavella JF, et al.: An update of epidemiologic studies of plutonium workers. *Health Phys* (in press) 1982.

52. Mancuso TF, Stewart A, Kneale GW: Radiation exposures of Hanford workers dying from cancer and other causes. *Health Phys* 1977; 33:369-385.

53. Kneale GW, Stewart A, Mancuso TF: Reanalysis of data relating to the Hanford study of the cancer risks of radiation effects. Int Symposium on Late Biological Effects Ionizing Radiat IAEA-SM-224/510, Vienna, March 13-17, 1978.

54. Anderson TW: Low-dose radiation (letter). *Lancet* 1978; 2:161.

55. Anderson TW: Radiation exposures of Hanford workers: A critique of the Mancuso, Stewart and Kneale report. *Health Phys* 1978; 35:743-750.

56. Mole RH 1978; Occupational exposure to ionising radiation (letter). Lancet 1978; 1:1155-1156.

57. Marks S, Gilbert ES, Breitenstein BD: Cancer mortality in Hanford workers. Symposium on Late Biological Effects Ionizing Radiat IAEA-SM-224, Vienna, March 13-17, 1978.

58. Gertz SM: Some major statistical comments on "Radiation exposures of Hanford workers dying from cancer and other causes", (letter). *Health Phys* 1978; 35:723-724.

59. Reissland JA: An Assessment of the Mancuso Study. National Radiological Protection Board, NRPB-R79, Harwell, Didcot, England, 1978.

60. Kneale GW, Stewart AM, Mancuso TF: Radiation exposures of Hanford workers dying from cancer and other causes (letter). *Health Phys* 1979; 36:87.

61. Mason TJ, McKay FW, Hoover R, et al.: Atlas of Cancer Mortality for U.S. Counties: 1950-1969 Epidemiology Branch, National Cancer Institute, DHEW Pub No (NIH) 75-780, 1975.

62. Bale WF, Shapiro JV: Radiation dosage to the lungs from randon and its daughter products. *Proceedings United Nations Conference on Peaceful Uses of Atomic Energy* Vol 13, New York, 1956. pp 233-236.

63. Wagoner JK, Archer VE, Carroll BE, et al.: Cancer mortality among U.S. uranium miners and millers 1950-1962. *J Natl Cancer Inst* 1964; 32:787-801.

64. Wagoner JK, Archer VE, Lundin FE, et al.: Radiation as the cause of lung cancer among uranium miners. *N Engl J Med* 1965; 273:181-188.

65. Lundin FE, William L, Smith EM: Mortality of uranium miners in relation to radiation exposure, hard-rock mining, and cigarette smoking — 1950 through September, 1967. *Health Phys* 1969; 16:571-578.

66. Lundin FE, Wagoner JK, Archer VE: Radon daughter exposure and respiratory cancer: Quantitative and temporal aspects. U.S. Dept Commerce Natl Tech Info Serv Pub No PB-204 871.

67. Saccomanno G, Saunders RP, Ellis H, et al.: Concentration of carcinoma or atypical cells in sputum. *Acta Cytol* 1963; 7:305-310.

68. Saccomanno G, Saunders RP, Archer VE, et al.: Cancer of the lung: The cytology of sputum prior to the development of carcinoma. *Acta Cytol* 1965; 9:413-423.

69. Saccomanno G, Archer VE, Auerbach O, et al.: Histologic types of lung cancer among uranium miners. *Cancer* 1971; 27:515–522.

70. Saccomanno G, Archer VE, Auerbach O, et al.: Susceptibility and resistance to environmental carcinogens in the development of carcinoma of the lung. *Human Pathol* 1973; 4:487–495.

71. Archer VE, Radford EP, Axelson O: Factors in exposure-response relationships of radon daughter injury. In: *Conference/Workshop on Lung Cancer Epidemiology. Industrial Applications of Sputum Cytology.* Golden: Colorado School of Mines Press, 1978. pp 324–367.

72. Radford EP: Radon daughters in the induction of lung cancer in underground miners. In: *Banbury Report 9: Quantification of Occupational Cancer,* Cold Spring Harbor Laboratory, New York: 1981. pp 151–163.

73. Hammond KR, Marvin BA: *Report to the Rocky Flats Monitoring Committee Concerning Scientists' Judgments of Cancer Risk.* Boulder: Univ. Colorado Center for Research on Judgment and Policy, 1981.

74. Anderson BF, Hammond KR, Berg J, et al.: *Second Report to the Rocky Flats Monitoring Committee Concerning Scientists' Judgments of Cancer Risk.* Univ Colorado School Medicine & Center for Research on Judgment Policy (Report No 233), 1981.

75. Doll R, Peto R: Cigarette smoking and bronchial carcinoma: Dose and time relationships among regular smokers and life long non-smokers. *J Epidemiol Community Health* 1978; 32:303–313.

76. Doll R, Hill AB: Mortality in relation to smoking: Ten years' observations of British doctors. *Brit Med J* 1964; 1:1399–1410, 1460–1467.

77. Hammond EC: Smoking in relation to the death rates of one million men and women. *Natl Cancer Inst Monogr* 1966; 19:127–204.

78. Kahn HA: The Dorn study of smoking and mortality among U.S. veterans: Report on eight and one-half years of observation. *Natl Cancer Inst Monogr* 1978; 19:1–37.

79. Archer VE, Gillam JD, Wagoner JK, et al.: Epidemiological studies of lung cancer among uranium miners of the Colorado plateau. In: *Conference/Workshop on Lung Cancer Epidemiology. Industrial Applications of Sputum Cytology.* Golden: Colorado School of Mines, 1978. pp 149–182.

80. Sutherland JV: Estimation of lung cancer risk from environmental exposure to airborn plutonium from the Rocky Flats Plant. *Proceedings of Special Workshop on Lung Dosimetry,* Radiation Research Society: Salt Lake City, 1982.

81. Barker CJ: Historical comparison: Colorado Department of Health/DOE Environmental Measurements Laboratory/Rocky Flats Plant: 1974–1978. Environmental Analysis Rocky Flats Plant ES-376-81-229, 1981.

82. Radford EP: Radon daughters in the induction of lung cancer in underground miners. In: *Banbury Report 9: Quantification of Occupational Cancer.* Cold Springs Harbor Laboratory, New York, 1981, pp 151–163.

23.

Nuclear Power and Its Alternatives

William R. Hendee

During the 1970s, two concerns evolved in the United States that promise to influence the course of American society in a profound manner. The first concern has been an awakening to the finite nature of the nation's energy resources. The second concern has been a recognition of the fragile character of the environment and the environmental impact of technologies associated with the recovery and utilization of energy resources. Conflicts between these concerns have resulted in a course for this society that promises to produce acute shortages of energy as well as significant environmental pollution by the end of the twentieth century, unless decisions are made now to alter the course of our society.

Most persons have some knowlege of the possible health and environmental hazards associated with the generation of electricity and the use of natural resources for the release of energy in other forms. On the other hand, few have considered the risks of running short of electricity and other forms of usable energy by the end of this decade. Risks associated with a shortage of energy resources are described as "downside risks" and have been categorized by Rossin[1] as follows.

Downside Risk 1: The Self-Fulfilling Prophecy. If the demand for energy resources such as electricity exceeds the supply within the next few years, industry will be forced to relocate where resources are available. That is, the availability of energy resources such as electricity could become a major influence on the job market, the industrial tax base, and the social stability of communities across the country. Communities lacking an adequate supply of electricity could encounter a downward spiral economically and socially that would be difficult to reverse.

Downside Risk 2: Government to the Rescue. With electricity and other energy resources in short supply, utilities probably would be accused of inadequate planning and expansion of capacity. If the shortage were severe enough, citizens probably would turn to government to operate the utilities and to build new power plants.

Downside Risk 3: Priorities and Allocations. If the demand for electricity were to exceed the supply, priorities for its use would have to be established. The allocation of electricity usage according to priorities is not an issue that can be resolved by private utilities; it is an issue that can be addressed only in the political arena, probably at the federal level. According to Rossin[1]:

> If the debate about nuclear energy is to deal with risks, the downside risks of electric energy shortage had better become a feature of it. If a free society is to arrive at an energy policy, its people need to be well aware of the downside risk of all of its options.

To satisfy the demand for electricity in the 1990s, utility officials estimate that 40,000 megawatts (MWe) should be added each year in the 1980s to the country's capacity to generate electrical power. At present, however, there is little financial incentive for utilities to invest in new plants for the generation of electricity. This lack of incentive is reflected in the following statistics:[2]

1. Since 1972, orders have been cancelled for 86 coal and nuclear generating plants totaling more than 85,000 MWe.
2. Delays averaging 40 months have been encountered by another 24 coal and nuclear power facilities amounting to more than 195,000 MWe originally planned for service in the early 1990s.
3. Over the past 2 years, only 20 net orders representing about 8,000 MWe have been placed for new coal-fired plants. No nuclear power plants have been ordered, and plans for plants totaling 25,000 MWe have been canceled.

Three solutions are apparent to the disparancy between the anticipated future need for electricity and the present commitment to build the power plants required to satisfy this need: (1) conservation; (2) development of alternative technologies for the generation of electricity; and (3) construction of more power plants that use conventional sources of energy. Each of these solutions is explored below, and probably all will be required to maintain the economic and social fabric of this country's society.

CONSERVATION

No matter how successful solutions 2 and 3 become, the conservation of energy resources will remain essential to the continuing viability of this country and its social and economic welfare. The essential nature of energy conservation has been recognized already; for example, from 1979 to 1980 oil imports were reduced by 20 percent.[3] Nevertheless, the United States still imported twice as much oil from OPEC countries in 1980 than in 1973.[4] With rigorous conservation measures, as much as a 25 percent reduction in the growth of energy consumption has been postulated for the remainder of the century. Even with this reduction, an increase in energy consumption over the next two decades has been predicted for the following reasons:[2]

1. The population of the United States will increase from 225 to 280 million.
2. The nation's workforce will increase from 105 to 130 million workers.
3. The number of households will increase from 80 to 115 million units.
4. The Gross National Product will expand from $2.6 to $4.7 trillion in 1980 U.S. dollars.

These factors are expected to increase the demand for energy from 76 quads[*] in 1980 to about 118 quads by the year 2000.

To satisfy the anticipated demand for energy by the year 2000, the supply of usable energy from various sources can be extrapolated to the turn of the century. This extrapolation, made by the Atomic Industrial Forum, has resulted in the following predictions:[2]

- *Petroleum:* New national sources and advanced techniques of recovery could maintain production at the current level of about 23 quads/year.
- *Natural gas:* In spite of new reservoirs and advanced methods of recovery, a slight reduction from current levels to about 17 quads/year is estimated.
- *Hydroelectric and geothermal:* Limited sites for additional development permit only a small increase to a level of about 3 quads.
- *Solar and renewable resources:* Problems of reliable technology and high cost probably will limit this energy source to an increase of about 5 quads in the year 2000.
- *Foreign fuels:* The implementation of import restrictions may limit this energy supply to perhaps 7 quads, about half its present level.

These sources total 55 quads, less than half the 118 quads predicted to be needed by the year 2000, even with a vigorous conservation program in effect.

ALTERNATIVE TECHNOLOGIES

A number of alternative technologies have been proposed as replacements for conventional sources of energy and as mechanisms to reduce this country's

---

[*]A quad is an amount of energy equivalent to that released by burning 172 million barrels of oil.

present dependence on oil imports from politically unstable countries. These technologies primarily use solar energy, biomass, and synthetic fuels, with somewhat less attention directed toward the use of wind, geothermal energy, and tidal power as energy sources. Fusion power might be included as well. Some of these sources of energy are proposed as environmentally clean and economically feasible, especially as decentralized energy sources, since they are distributed over the landscape. In most cases, however, the distributed nature of these energy sources is their major limitation.

Although wind, geothermal, and tidal power have received some attention as desirable alternative energy sources, their contribution to the supply of energy in the year 2000 is estimated at no more than 1 percent of the total supply of energy.[5] This small contribution is primarily attributable to the limited availability of suitable sites in the case of geothermal energy and to the distributed nature of the power source in the case of wind and tidal power. In addition, the rather primitive state of current technology and the high cost of energy-conversion devices impose severe limitations on the use of these energy resources. Although "soft" technologies (i.e., decentralized and nonpolluting sources of energy), such as geothermal, wind, and tidal power might have some desirable features, their net contribution to this country's energy supply by the year 2000 will probably be negligible.

A similar skepticism surrounds fusion power in terms of its contribution to the supply of energy for the nation by the year 2000. In spite of increases in plasma temperatures and confinement times over the past few years, the realization of fusion power appears further away today than it was 20 years ago, when it was heralded as the ultimate energy resource. Furthermore, the public often equates fusion power with fission power, and supporters of this technology could encounter a hostile public similar to that currently experienced by advocates of fission power.[6,7] This inappropriate linkage further diminishes the likelihood of fusion power as a significant source of energy by the year 2000.

Solar energy is one soft technology that is expected to contribute significantly to the country's energy needs by the turn of the century. This contribution is expected to be primarily in the decentralized form of space and water heating in residences. Together with wood, solar energy should supply about 5 quads to the nation's energy supply in the year 2000. More extensive use of solar is limited by the distributed nature of this energy source and by the expense of installing solar collectors and storage media. Technologic breakthroughs in conversion and storage devices for solar energy could enhance its contribution, but the distributed character of this energy source will ultimately limit the contribution to considerably less than 10 percent of the nation's energy supply.

The conversion of biomass and synthetic fuels to usable sources of energy is so hypothetical that it is difficult to predict the final contribution of these materials to the nation's energy supply. Two limitations in these sources are already apparent, however: synthetic fuels are likely to be expensive and conversion processes for biomass produce considerable pollution. To discount these materials as significant sources of energy by the turn of the century is probably the most prudent posture at this time.

CONVENTIONAL ENERGY SOURCES

Although conservation and alternate technologies will contribute significantly to the country's energy supply, the bulk of its energy will continue to be provided by conventional sources of power in the year 2000. As described earlier, national reserves of petroleum and natural gas are expected to remain relatively constant over the next 20 years, contributing about 40 quads by century's end. Hydro- and geothermal power, solar energy and renewable resources should add perhaps another 8 quads to the energy supply, and foreign fuels may provide about 7 quads if federal programs for import reduction are implemented. Collectively, these sources amount to about 55 quads of energy, less than half the demand of 118 quads anticipated for the year 2000, even with vigorous measures of energy conservation. The remainder of the energy supply must come from either coal and nuclear, or from the importation of foreign fuels at a level above that projected by federal import quotas. Coal and nuclear are utilized more efficiently as centralized energy sources for the production of electricity. In 1980, approximately one-third of the nation's energy supply was used to produce electricity; by the turn of the century, this fraction is expected to increase to about half. This increase is consistent with an increased dependence on coal and nuclear as principal resources for energy production.

Demonstrated reserves of recoverable coal could satisfy the present demand for energy in the United States for well over 300 years.[2] If the rate of increase in coal usage over the next 18 years were to be twice the historical average, then the contribution of coal to the nation's energy supply could reach 45 quads by the year 2000. However, the utilization of coal is hazardous to workers who mine and transport the coal as well as to members of the public exposed to the transportation process and to the pollutants released when coal is burned. The hazards of coal utilization compared with the hazards of uranium for the production of electricity are demonstrated in the following statistics:[5 8-13]

- *Per billion megawatt-hours (MWh) of electricity*, the cost in fatal mining accidents is 189 lives in coal mining and 18 lives in uranium mining.
- *Per million MWh of electricity*, injuries cost 1545 disability-days for

coal mining and 157 disability-days for uranium mining.

- *Per billion MWh of electricity*, there are 1000 deaths by black lung disease among coal miners and 20 deaths by excess lung cancers among uranium miners.
- *Per thousand megawatt-years (MWy) of electricity*, the amount of fuel required is 38,000 rail cars of coal resulting in 100 transportation deaths. For nuclear power, the fuel required is six truckloads of uranium, probably resulting in no transportation deaths.
- *Radioactive releases from a coal-fired power plant* pose 410 times the health threat of radioactive emissions from a nuclear plant of identical size. (Some investigators argue that this estimated difference is too large, but virtually all agree that radioactivity from coal-fired plants is more hazardous than that from nuclear plants.)
- *Per thousand MWy of electricity*, 20–100 excess deaths occur each year from respiratory diseases induced by air pollution from coal-fired power plants. (For nuclear plants, fewer than 1, and probably 0, excess deaths occur each year from respiratory diseases induced by air pollution.)

With the addition of 45 quads of energy from coal to the 55 quads of energy available from petroleum, natural gas, solar, hydro, geothermal, renewable sources, and foreign fuels, a balance of only 18 quads remains to satisfy the anticipated energy needs of this country in the year 2000. This balance could easily be supplied by nuclear power. In fact, available reactor technology combined with known sources of uranium in this country could replace the entire amount of energy supplied by domestic coal, oil, and gas by the year 2000. To meet even the 18 quad requirement by the turn of the century, however, utilities in the 1980s must order as much new nuclear-generating capacity as that already operating or under construction. To achieve this nuclear capacity, and to achieve the 118-quad energy requirement anticipated for the year 2000, many new facilities will be required for the generation of electricity. These new facilities must provide approximately 600,000 MWe of generating capacity over the next two decades, an amount about equal to that presently in service in the nation's total electrical power network. An expanded electrical power program of this magnitude would require an investment of more than $500 billion, an amount about twice the net worth of all electrical power plants currently in operation or under construction.

Deployment of new facilities for the generation of electricity over the next 18 years will require the removal of present obstacles to expansion of the country's electrical network. Among these obstacles are the following:

- Poor investment potential of electric utilities

- Poor return on investment in new facilities for electricity generation
- Unpredictable, expensive, and agonizingly slow licensing procedures
- Above all, the lack of development of a prudent, pragmatic energy program by the country's public and political leaders

For nuclear power to contribute significantly to the alleviation of demands for increased electricity by the year 2000, a further obstacle must be overcome, namely the present nuclear phobia of the American public. This phobia can be addressed only through public education leading to a balanced perspective of the benefits and hazards of nuclear power compared with those of alternate sources of energy and to the risks associated with an insufficient supply of energy in a few years. Also to be considered in a public education effort should be the precarious and capricious nature of this country's continued reliance on energy sources imported from politically unstable countries, as well as the risk this importation poses for the nation's economic, social and military security.

As decribed by the Atomic Industrial Forum[2]:

Considering the decade or more required to place a new coal or nuclear generating unit in service, however, the future is now; without ensuring expansion of power producing capability today, major and chronic shortages of electricity are inevitable in the years ahead.

And, as emphasized by Mills[4]:

The key elements for a secure United States energy policy are sensible and economic conservation in concert with, not in competition with, sensible coal and nuclear development.

REFERENCES

1. Rossin AD: Energy shortage: The downside risks. *Public Util Fortnightly,* July 17, 1980, 46.
2. *Nuclear Power Information.* Washington DC, Atomic Industrial Forum, 1981.
3. *Monthly Energy Review:* US Department of Energy, March 1981.
4. Mills M: *Recharging America: One Alternative to Oil Imports.* Washington, DC Atomic Industrial Forum, 1981.
5. Beckmann, P: *The Health Hazards of Not Going Nuclear.* Boulder, Golem Press, 1976.
6. Hebert JA, Shikiar, R. Perception of fusion power: Topical report. Battelle Human Affairs Research Report 411/81/006. Seattle, Battelle, 1981.
7. Goldstein, C: Perceptions of fusion power: A backward glance into the future.

Washington DC, Atomic Industrial Forum, 1981.

8. Lave LB, Freiburg LC: Health effects of electricity generation from coal, oil and nuclear fuel. *Nuclear Safety* 1973; 14:409.

9. Wilson, R: Energy Conference, Center for Science, Technology and Political Thought, Denver, June 1974.

10. Rose DJ, Walsh PW, Leskovjan LL: Nuclear power *vis-a-vis* its alternatives, chiefly coal. In Beckmann P (ed): *The Health Hazards of Not Going Nuclear.* Boulder, Golem Press, 1976.

11. Rollins MR, Williams RW, Meyer W: Estimates of the economic effects of a five year nuclear moratorium. University of Missouri, 1975.

12. Wilson R, Jones WJ: *Energy, Ecology and the Environment.* New York, Academic Press, 1974.

13. Lave LB, Seskin E: An analysis of the association between U.S. mortality and air pollution. University of Pittsburgh report, 1971.

24.

Management of Radioactive Wastes

William R. Hendee

The disposal of radioactive wastes is perhaps the most controversial and least understood aspect of the use of nuclear materials in generating electrical power, the investigation of biochemical processes through tracer kinetics, and the diagnosis and treatment of disease. In the siting of nuclear power facilities, the disposal of radioactive wastes is invariably posed as the ultimate unanswerable question. In the fall of 1979, biochemical and physiologic research employing radioactive tracers was threatened with a slowdown resulting from temporary closure of sites for disposal of low-level radioactive wastes (LLW). Radioactive pharmaceuticals used extensively for diagnosis and treatment of human disease have increased dramatically in price, partly as a result of the escalating cost of disposing of radioactive wastes created during production of the labeled pharmaceuticals. These problems have resulted in identification of the disposal of LLW as the most pressing issue in the entire scheme of management of hazardous wastes. How this issue as well as the separate issue of disposal of high-level radioactive wastes (HLW) are being addressed at both national and state levels is the subject of this chapter.

High-level radioactive wastes are produced by the nuclear weapons industry and by public utilities that operate nuclear power reactors for the generation of electricity. Over the past 35+ years, the nuclear weapons industry has produced more than 80×10^6 gallons of HLW. Currently, these wastes are held in temporary storage at various government reservations across the country, where they await implementation of a national program for HLW disposal. Awaiting the same solution are HLW produced in nuclear power reactors. These wastes, primarily in the form of spent nuclear fuel containing residual uranium, newly created plutonium, and radioactive fission products, are stored temporarily in deep pools of water on-site at the power reactors. About 30 tons of spent fuel are created annually in a 1000-megawatt (MW) nuclear power reactor.

Until 1977, spent fuel from nuclear power reactors was stored under the assumption that chemical reprocessing of the spent fuel to recover the residual uranium and newly created plutonium would be technologically and economically feasible by the 1980s. Chemical processing would involve dissolving the spent fuel in nitric acid to form a solution from which the uranium and plutonium could be extracted for eventual fabrication into fresh fuel. High-level radioactive wastes from the extraction process would then be converted into a dry solid state, calcined to fine particles, fused into a melted glass mixture (vitrification), and solidified into thick glass rods sealed within metal canisters. The canisters would be encased in large concrete blocks for permanent storage in a stable geologic formation 1000–2000 feet below the earth's surface. Ten canisters, each about 14 inches in diameter by 12 feet long, would contain all the HLW from reprocessed spent fuel produced during 1 year of operation of a 1000-MW power reactor. About 25,000 canisters, occupying a volume of approximately 320,000 ft^3, would contain the solidified reprocessing wastes from all commercial power reactors operating through the end of the century in the United States.[1]

The ideal geologic formations for permanent storage of HLW appear to be salt formations. These formations have been geologically stable for hundreds of millions of years and have a diminishingly small possibility of becoming contaminated with groundwater that might return radioactive wastes to the environment should the vitrified wastes ever become permeable to environmental influences. Other candidates for permanent storage include granite, argillaceous clays and volcanic tuff. All four possibilities for permanent storage are readily available in the United States. Germany has implemented permanent storage of radioactive wastes in an abandoned salt mine, and France and Sweden have indicated that they consider the process safe with virtually insignificant risks and negligible effects on the health of the public.[2]

In April 1977, a presidential policy was announced to reduce the risk of proliferation of nuclear weapons. As part of this policy, an indefinite deferral was imposed on the chemical reprocessing of spent nuclear fuel. Consequently, permanent storage of spent nuclear fuel itself, rather than the HLW generated by reprocessing this fuel, must now be considered. The procedure for treating the waste will remain essentially unchanged, but the volume of HLW will be increased about eightfold. Many people believe that the policy of indefinite deferral of reprocessing spent fuel eventually will be rescinded perhaps by the current administration in Washington DC.

In April 1977, the President also established an Interagency Review Group on nuclear waste management. In March 1979 the final report of the Review Group was released with plans for the selection and licensing of a permanent repository for the storage of HLW. In February 1980, the President announced preliminary guidelines for a new national program for radioactive waste management to be developed by the Department of Energy, other federal agencies, and state and local governments.

In response to the presidential directive, the Department of Energy has announced plans to identify three specific locations for intensive study as permanent storage sites for HLW. Two of the sites will be on government reservations and the third site will be a salt formation. Drilling of exploratory shafts at these sites is anticipated by 1983, and by 1985 a test facility for HLW storage is planned. A final repository for HLW is scheduled to become operational sometime between 1987 and 2000.

The management of HLW is technologically feasible, and problems with its implementation appear to be more political than technical in nature. Demonstration of progress by the Department of Energy in the selection and feasibility study of a potential site might enhance the political and public acceptance of a HLW repository. Recission of the indefinite deferral on reprocessing spent nuclear fuel would also help by significantly reducing the volume of HLW to be managed.

To be classified as LLW, radioactive materials must satisfy three criteria:

1. They must not be HLW.
2. They must contain <10 nCi/g of transuranic nuclides.
3. They must not be mine or mill tailings.

Low-level wastes can be solid, liquid, or gaseous and include routine wastes from research establishments, medical institutions, industrial facilities, and power reactors contaminated with small quantities of radioactivity. Disposal of these wastes is by burial in near-surface disposal sites.

In the United States, six disposal sites have been used for commercial disposal of LLW, and three are operating today. The three commercial sites that are now closed are located at West Valley, New York; Maxey Flats, Kentucky; and Sheffield, Illinois. The West Valley site was closed because inadequate drainage caused disposal trenches to fill with rainwater and overflow. The Maxey Flats site was closed by the operator because the state imposed such a high surcharge for waste disposal that continued operation was uneconomical. The site at Sheffield closed when it reached its licensed capacity for waste disposal and expansion was opposed by state authorities. The three sites that currently are operational are located at Barnwell, South Carolina; Hanford, Washington; and Beatty, Nevada.

In 1980, 90,928 m³ of LLW was buried in the three disposal sites commercially available.[3] The Barnwell site received 54,725 m³ (or 59 percent) of this waste, with the remainder distributed beween the Hanford (24,824 m³, or 27 percent) and Beatty (12,732 m³, or 14 percent) sites. Slightly more than half the waste was generated by nuclear power plants, with industry and medical and research facilities contributing about equally to the remainder. New York, South Carolina, Pennsylvania, and Illinois were the largest producers of LLW, accounting for close to 40 percent of the total volume of LLW handled for the year. Nevada and Washington, two states that provide disposal sites, collectively contributed less than 2 percent of the total LLW buried in the three disposal sites. The volume of radioactive waste generated at facilities in Colorado was less then 1 percent of the national total, as was the volume of waste generated by Arizona, New Mexico, Utah, Nevada, and Wyoming, with which Colorado is negotiating a compact agreement (see below).

Beginning in 1982, the disposal site at Barnwell has been limited to 34,000 m³ of LLW, or about 40 percent of the current national total. This reduction in waste handling capacity at Barnwell has both expanded the waste-disposal burden on the two remaining sites and increased the cost and hazard of transporting radioactive wastes over long distances. In November 1980, Washington voters enacted Initiative 383, preventing the disposal of non-medical LLW at Hanford that originates from facilities outside the state of Washington. Although this initiative was ruled unconstitutional in June 1981 and will not be enforced, the ruling of unconstitutionality has been appealed by the state. In the fall of 1980, regulatory authorities in Nevada attempted to prevent renewal of the license of Nuclear Engineering Company (now U.S. Ecology Inc.) to operate the Beatty, Nevada, disposal site. Although this attempt proved unsuccessful, it resulted in inspection regulations and fees that have increased the cost and paperwork associated with the disposal of LLW at the Beatty site. Currently, the cost of disposal of LLW varies from $200 to $300 per 55 gallon drum, depending on the type of waste and the distance it has to be transported.

With the commissioning of additional nuclear power plants and the ever-expanding use of radioactive materials in research, medicine, and industry, the volume of LLW is expected to increase at a rate greater than 10 percent per year over the next few years. It has been estimated that by 1990, the rate of generation of LLW will be as high as 183,700 m³/year.[4] This estimate does not include the large volumes of radioactive waste associated with the decommissioning of nuclear power plants, a process that could attain major importance by the year 2000.

In August 1980, a task force report was released by the National Governors Association that addressed the issue of the disposal of low-level radioactive waste.[5] This report, subsequently endorsed by the National Conference of State Legislatures and the State Planning Council, divided the United States into six regions, with one disposal site for LLW to be located centrally in each region. Six disposal sites probably would provide adequate disposal capacity for LLW through the year 2000, and the sites could be positioned strategically to minimize the cost of transporting wastes. The Nuclear Regulatory Commission has issued proposed regulations governing the classification of radioactive wastes and the licensure of new shallow land burial disposal sites.[6] Problems associated with implementation of new disposal sites for LLW are more political than technical in nature and will have to be approved through the political process, with all its subjectivity and uncertainty.

The political aspects of the LLW issue were aided in December 1980 by congressional passage of the Low Level Waste Policy Act (P.L. 96-573). This act incorporates the recommendations of the report of the National Governors Association Task Force on Low-Level Radioactive Waste Disposal as well as the suggestions developed by a task force of the Department of Energy, with EG & G Idaho serving as the lead agency.[7] An important feature of P.L. 96-573 is the assignment of responsibility to each individual state for the management of LLW within the state. The act also encouraged the development of disposal facilities on a regional basis as a result of compact agreements negotiated among individual states.

In response to the Low Level Waste Policy Act, representatives from governors' offices have been meeting on a regional basis to develop strategies for solving the LLW disposal problem. A compact agreement has already been enacted involving Oregon, Washington, and Idaho, and others are in different stages of completion. In the Southwest, a draft compact has been written for Colorado, New Mexico, Arizona, Nevada, Utah, and Wyoming. This document was discussed at length in November 1981, at a meeting in Denver attended by representatives from each of the states involved and sponsored by the Western Interstate Energy Board, the state of Colorado, the National Conference of State Legislatures, and the Western Council of the Council of State Governments. Suggestions emanating from this discussion were incorporated into a revision of the compact to be considered by the legislatures in each of the states participating in the compact. In Colorado, Wyoming and New Mexico the revised compact agreement has already been approved by the state legislature, and the Southwest compact agreement has been submitted to Congress for ratification.

Low-level radioactive waste is probably one of the most benign and easily managed hazardous wastes produced as a by-product of a highly scientific and industrial society. Although its management might be readily available from a technical viewpoint, the political character of the issue is far more intractable. For this reason, legislators and representatives of state executive offices will need all the wisdom within reach as they grapple with the issues of managing low-level radioactive wastes.

REFERENCES

1. *Nuclear Power Information.* Washington, DC, Atomic Industrial Forum, 1981.
2. Commonwealth Edison Company Notes, May 1979.
3. Levin, GB: Low-Level radioactive waste management in the U.S.: A proving ground. *Nuclear News* 1971; 72.

4. US Department of Energy: Report to Congress on Public Law 96-573, July 21, 1981.

5. *National Governors Association Task Force on Low-Level Radioactive Waste Disposal.* Final Report. 1980.

6. Licensing requirement for land disposal facilities for radioactive waste. Title 10, *Code of Federal Regulations,* Chapter 61.

7. EG & G Idaho: Managing low-level radioactive waste-approach, LLWMP-1. 1980.

25.

Radiation and Political Fallout of Three Mile Island

Donald B. Hess
William R. Hendee

Originally only one nuclear power reactor was intended for Three Mile Island (TMI), a small piece of land on the Susquehanna River in southeastern Pennsylvania. The second reactor, Unit 2, was sited on TMI not by design but as a result of a labor dispute. It was Unit 2 that on March 28, 1979 produced the most publicized incident ever involving a nuclear power plant.

In the late 1960s, a nuclear power reactor was under construction on TMI under the general supervision of Metropolitan Edison Company (Met Ed). To coordinate the substantial capital expenditures required for construction of Unit 1 and other power plants, Met Ed had combined with Jersey Central Power and Light and with the Pennsylvania Electric Company to form the General Public Utilities Corporation (GPU). Under the GPU rubric, Jersey Power and Light also was supervising the construction of two nuclear power plants in Oyster Creek, New Jersey. Construction was nearly complete on one unit, and the second unit was well into the planning stage, when a labor dispute arose involving a demand of 1 percent of total construction costs as a bonus for initiation of construction.[1] This demand was rejected, and GPU transferred the second reactor to TMI under the supervision of Met Ed, somewhat to the consternation of the latter, since the transferred reactor differed significantly from the unit previously sited on TMI.

Construction at TMI proceeded uneventfully, and Unit 2 was subjected to its first criticality test on March 27, 1978, 1 year and a day before its appointment with infamy. Over the following months, a number of minor problems were identified and corrected, and Unit 2 entered the commercial network of electrical power plants 25 hours before the close of 1978.[2]

Three months later, at 4 o'clock A.M. on March 28, 1979, Unit 2 was operating uneventfully at 97 percent peak power.[3] Water in the primary coolant loop was heated under high pressure in the reactor core. By circulating this water through a heat exchanger, the heat was transferred to

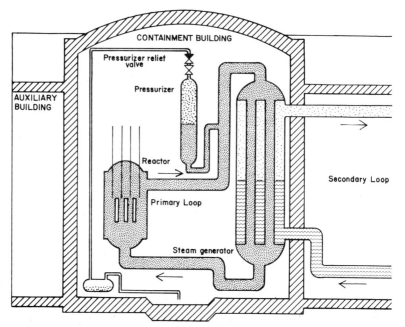

Figure 1. Heating and cooling processes in TMI-2. The Primary Loop carries heat from the reactor to the steam generator and returns to the reactor. In the Secondary Loop, heat is received from the primary loop and used to produce steam to drive the turbine generator. Heat from the spent steam is transferred to the condenser cooling loop and carried to the cooling tower, where it is discharged into the atmosphere. (From Barker B (ed): Prelude: The accident at Three Mile Island. *Electric Power Res Inst J* June 1980; 7–13.)

water in the secondary coolant loop, which in turn was converted to steam used to drive turbines to generate eletrical power. In the condenser, steam leaving the turbine was cooled to water, with the liberated heat transferred to the cooling tower by circulating water. The heating and cooling processes for primary and secondary coolant systems are depicted in Figure 1.

For a number of days, operators of Unit 2 had been aware of a slow leak of coolant from the primary loop, probably through a malfunctioning pressure relief valve (PRV). To compensate for the slow leak, water was added to the primary loop by the operators to maintain the pressure in the primary loop at a normal level. The malfunctioning valve causing a slow loss of coolant was not a major problem in itself; however, it did contribute to incorrect temperature readings in the drain pipe past the pressure relief valve. These readings later camouflaged a more serious loss of coolant.[3]

A second problem also existed on the morning of March 28, 1979. Two valves in the auxiliary feedwater system had been left closed after routine

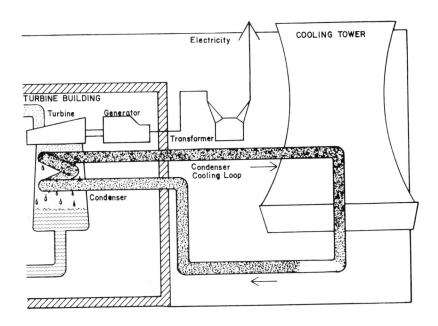

maintenance 2 days earlier. Operators of Unit 2 were not aware of the existence of this problem.

A third problem that developed on the morning in question was a series of events that in common parlance have become known as "The TMI Accident." For hours the operators had been attempting under remote control to transfer spent resins from the polishers to the resin regeneration tank. These resins are used to purify the water in the secondary coolant system, and they are transferred periodically to the regeneration tank for restoration. On March 28, however, the transfer process became obstructed, automatically causing the condensate pumps to shut off. Immediately, the main feedwater pumps followed suit according to design, causing a complete loss of feedwater to the steam generators. In response, the main turbine switched off, and at precisely 4:00:37 the TMI accident had begun (Fig. 2).[4]

To compensate for the loss of coolant to the steam generators when the main feedwater pumps stopped working, the auxiliary feedwater pumps were activated. As noted earlier, however, valves in the auxiliary feedwater circuit had been left closed, so that none of the auxiliary feedwater could reach the steam generators. With no water flowing in the secondary coolant loop, heat could not be transferred across the heat exchangers, and the temperature of the primary water began to rise. This rise in temperature led to an increase in pressure in the primary coolant loop.

The pressure of the primary coolant increased until it reached the level

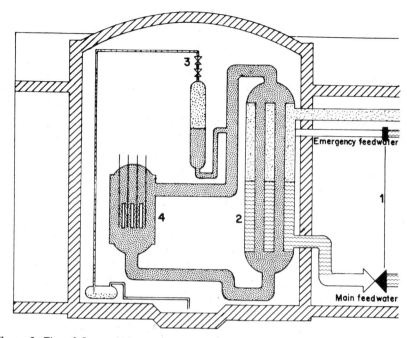

Figure 2. Time 0 Seconds.[1] As a result of maintenance work, the main feedwater pumps trip. Emergency feedwater flow is blocked by two valves that inadvertently had been left closed sometime during the previous two days. [2] When feedwater flow stops, heat removal from the primary system decreases. [3] At 3 seconds, a relief valve on the pressurizer opens to reduce momentary overpressure, but then fails to close when the pressure drops. Operators are not aware that the valve is open. [4] The reactor shuts down at 8 seconds. (From Barker B (ed): Prelude: The accident at Three Mile Island. *Electric Power Res Inst J* June 1980; 7-13.)

at which the pressure relief valve was set to open. Because of the first problem, this valve was already partly open, and the rising pressure caused it to open completely. However, the pressure was increasing so rapidly that the valve did not serve as an effective deterrent to the rising pressure. Instead, the pressure in the primary coolant loop continued to increase until it reached a level at which the reactor "scrammed." In the scram process, control rods drop into the reactor core to halt the fission process, immediately terminating the release of fission energy in the core of the reactor. Although the scram process reduced the generation of heat in the reactor core, it did not stop it completely; decay of radioactive products in the fuel rods continued to release heat at a rate of about 6 percent of that released while fission was occurring.[4] At this moment in the history of the TMI accident, the incident was 8 seconds old.

With reduced production of heat and an open pressure relief valve, the pressure in the primary coolant loop subsided rapidly. This reduction in pressure should have caused the pressure relief valve to close, thereby preventing any further loss of coolant in the primary loop.[4] As noted earlier, however, the pressure relief valve was not operating properly, causing it to remain open even though the pressure had dropped and a light on the reactor control panel indicated that the valve was closed. The continued loss of coolant through the open valve, and the operators' unawareness that this event was occurring, constituted the first major error in the TMI episode.

In the pressurizer portion of the primary coolant loop, a large bubble of steam is present to maintain the pressure at an equilibrium level. As the temperature of the coolant increases and decreases within limits, the steam bubble contracts and expands to keep the pressure on a relatively even keel. With the pressure-relief valve open, however, steam rapidly escaped from the primary coolant loop and was replaced by liquid coolant from the core coolant system. This gradual exchange of liquid coolant for steam eventually resulted in a pressurizer full of water, a condition described as "going solid."[5] In the solid condition, there is little tolerance of acute changes in pressure, and a high pressure spike can rupture the core coolant system.[4]

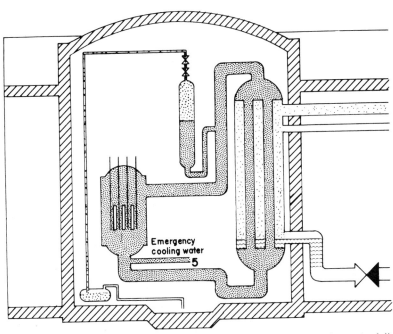

Figure 3. Time 2 minutes. [5] Pressure in the primary system continues to fall and triggers automatic injection of emergency cooling water into the core. At 5 minutes this process is throttled by the operators, who believe the system is overfilled with water because the pressurizer is full. (From Barker B (ed): Prelude: The accident at Three Mile Island. *Electric Power Res Inst J* June 1980; 7–13.)

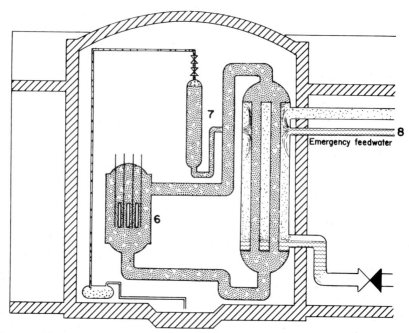

Figure 4. Time 5 minutes, 30 seconds. [6] Water in the core begins to boil. [7] Increasing steam volume forces water into the pressurizer. The high water level in the pressurizer continues to mislead operators into believing the primary system is overfilled. [8] Operators discover the closed valves in the emergency feedwater lines and open them at 8 minutes. (From Barker B (ed): Prelude: The accident at Three Mile Island. *Electric Power Res Inst J* June 1980; 7–13.)

As the pressure dropped in the primary coolant system, high-pressure injection pumps automatically began to inject water directly into the system to maintain the coolant pressure at the desired level. This stage in the TMI incident is described in Figure 3. In response, the pressure once again began to rise in the primary coolant system. Sensing that the rising pressure might signify that the reactor was going solid, the operators stopped the high-pressure injection pumps. This decision constituted the second major error in the TMI incident, and occured 5 minutes into the incident. Actually, to the contrary, the primary coolant system was not solid at this time; steam bubbles still existed in the system because of the open pressure-relief valve (PRV (Fig. 4). The presence of these bubbles went undetected, however, primarily because of the abnormal character of pressure readings in the primary coolant loop. For example, the operators had been taught that the level of coolant in the pressurizer should rise and fall in synchrony with the pressure in the primary coolant loop. In the early morning hours of March 28, 1979, however, these two parameters moved in opposite directions as the level of

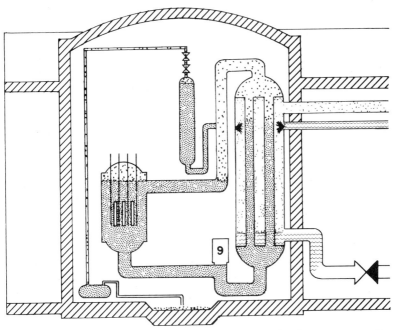

Figure 5 Time 1 hour, 40 minutes. Insufficient water remains for proper operation of reactor cooling pumps. Pumps begin to vibrate excessively. [9] The last two pumps are shut off at 1 hour, 40 minutes. (From Barker B (ed): Prelude: The accident at Three Mile Island. *Electric Power Res Inst J* June 1980; 7–13.)

coolant in the pressurizer rose and the pressure in the primary coolant dropped because of the presence of steam bubbles in the loop. Although this behavior implies an open pressure relief valve, this implication was not recognized by the operators; their training and experience did not encompass erratic behavior of this type.[5]

As the temperature of the steam-water mixture rose in the primary coolant loop, the reactor coolant pumps exhibited increased vibration, and the operators became increasingly concerned about seal failures in the pumps. To prevent these failures, the operators finally deactivated the reactor coolant pumps at 1 hour and 40 minutes into the incident (Figure 5). This action essentially sealed the fate of TMI-2, as now there was almost no conduction of heat from the reactor core.[3] Although auxiliary feedwater eventually was established to the primary coolant loop, it was of little help in preventing succeeding events in the saga. Heat from the reactor core further vaporized the water in the primary coolant loop and initiated the process of uncovering the fuel rods in the core of the reactor. In addition, the high temperature and the superheated steam environment led to a chemical reaction between the steam and the zirconium alloy ("zircalloy") cladding and

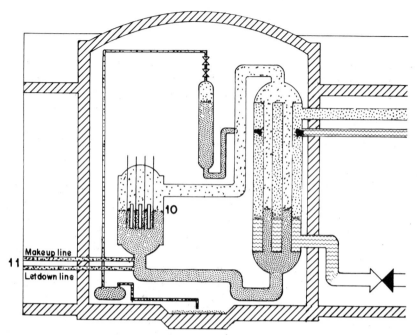

Figure 6. Time 2 hours. (10) After the pumps are shut off, the core begins to overheat and the fuel cladding begins to fail. (11) A small fraction of the radioactive gases from the fuel travel with the primary system water to the auxiliary building through the piping (letdown line) of the level control and purification system. (From Barker B (ed): Prelude: The accident at Three Mile Island. *Electric Power Res Inst J* June 1980; 7–13.)

a leakage of radioactivity from the fuel rods into the primary coolant loop and, later, into an auxiliary building (Fig. 6). It was this radioactivity that eventually was vented to the environment as approximately 10 MCi of xenon-133 and 15 Ci of iodine-131.[4]

The chemical reaction between the fuel rod cladding and the super-heated steam created a situation that was viewed by officials of the Nuclear Regulatory Commission (NRC) as potentially the most hazardous event in the entire TMI scenario. This situation was the release of a large quantity of hydrogen during the reaction process. In part, this hydrogen became trapped in the containment vessel surrounding the reactor core, creating a bubble that, in the opinion of NRC representatives, might combine with oxygen and explode. The NRC representatives surmised that such an explosion might breach the integrity of the containment vessel and release large quantities of radionuclides into the containment building. At the time of the accident, it was thought that sufficient oxygen might be present in the containment vessel to cause an explosion as a result of the radiolysis of water vapor by the intense

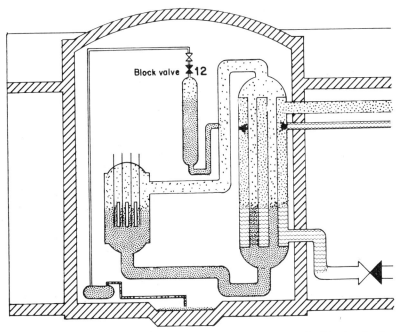

Figure 7. Time 2 hours, 18 minutes. [12] The operator closes the block valve to stop the flow through the open pressurizer relief valve. The loss of primary system water is stopped. (From Barker B (ed): Prelude: The accident at Three Mile Island. *Electric Power Res Inst J* June 1980; 7–13.)

radiation present in the reactor core. In retrospect, it is now relatively certain that too little oxygen was present in the vessel to cause an explosion upon combination with hydrogen. This insight was not available at the time of the incident, however, and the possibility of a H_2–O_2 explosion within the containment vessel was described as such not only to the people involved in the incident, but also to the news media, and, therefore, to the general public.[5]

At 2 hours and 18 minutes into the incident, the operators finally recognized the possibility of an open pressure relief valve (Fig. 7), and the flow of coolant was terminated through this leg of the primary coolant loop.[5] This action prevented any further loss of coolant and was the first human step toward recovery from the incident. After this action, a number of attempts were made to remove heat from the core coolant system. Finally, 16 hours after the incident had started, a reactor coolant pump was started and operated manually and the system began to approach stability. Two hours after the first pump was started, a second reactor coolant pump was started and added to the capacity to bring the reactor manually into equilibrium.[3]

In retrospect, the TMI incident did not compromise the physical health and well-being of anyone in the immediate vicinity of the plant; however, some claims of emotional and psychological stress have been levied. Among the lessons learned from the incident have been the need for improved engineering design of a power reactor from the systems approach and increased emphasis on the training of operators to enable them to respond appropriately, and not just "by the book." These lessons are reflected in many improvements made since the incident, including the creation of the Nuclear Safety Analysis Center and the Institute for Nuclear Power Operations.[5] Perhaps the most valuable lesson evolving from the TMI incident has been identification of the extensive overlapping of jurisdictional authority of a variety of government agencies at both the federal and state levels.

At the time of the incident, the federal plan designed to respond to nuclear emergencies was the Interagency Radiological Assistance Plan (IRAP). This plan was more a memorandum of understanding than an actual emergency response plan and was to be conducted by the descendants of the Atomic Energy Commission (AEC), the Nuclear Regulatory Commission (NRC), and the Department of Energy (DOE). During the incident, however, it quickly became apparent that some confusion existed concerning which agency was responsible for initiating the plan. Furthermore, a number of agencies believed that IRAP had been superseded by the Federal Disaster Assistance Administration (FDAA), and that coordination through the aegis of IRAP no longer applied. The FDAA itself believed that it was responsible for coordinating the emergency response to TMI at the federal level, since it had been created to assist state and local governments in times of declared disaster. Also involved in coordination of the federal response to TMI was the Federal Preparedness Agency (FPA), even though this agency was designed primarily to be involved more in wartime planning than in peacetime disasters. Another federal agency that had self-imposed jurisdictional authority during the TMI incident was the Defense Civil Preparedness Agency (DCPA).[1] These organizations were among the more prominent but not the only federal agencies involved in the TMI incident; a number of others became involved at different times after initiation of the incident. The result of this overlapping jurisdictional authority was a stream of confusing and conflicting orders and suggestions that contributed more to the problem than to the solution.

As the principal federal agency involved in nuclear power operations, the NRC was notified within a few hours of the beginning of the TMI incident. In response, the NRC activated the Incident Response Action Center in Bethesda, Maryland, to monitor the incident and to intercede wherever necessary in the management of the situation. In addition, the regional NRC office in King of Prussia, Pennsylvania, dispatched an emergency response team to the TMI site to work with officials of Met Ed in handling the technical aspects of the incident.[4] Interactions of the NRC representatives among themselves and with officials of Met Ed added further confusion, which ultimately contributed to the "decision-by-crisis" atmosphere of TMI.

At the state level, the Pennsylvania Emergency Management Agency (PEMA) was notified about 3 hours after initiation of the incident and was continuously involved in the development of evacuation plans for the populace around TMI from that time on. The Pennsylvania Bureau of Radiation Protection (PBRP) served as a resource to PEMA; its recommendations were passed through PEMA to the lieutenant governor as well as to officials of the counties in the vicinity of TMI. The lieutenant governor relayed information to the governor, who ultimately was responsible for issuing orders for evacuation pending declaration of a state of emergency by an appropriate federal agency.[1]

One and a half days after the beginning of the TMI incident, the secretary of health of Pennsylvania received a phone message from an official of the National Institute of Occupational Safety and Health. The official expressed concern over the condition of the reactor and that the condition might become uncontrollable. What was said next is somewhat unclear. According to the secretary, the official stated that he had consulted with the Bureau of Radiological Health of the federal Food and Drug Administration and that this consultation and his own experience mandated that the governor issue an order for evacuation of counties near TMI.[1] The governor was wise enough to defer action on this mandate, although later he recommended evacuation of pregnant women and children within a radius of 5 miles around TMI. The NRC at first vacillated and then recommended a general evacuation of the populace within a 10-mile radius of the TMI site.[2]

With all the government agencies involved in the TMI incident, it is little wonder that jurisdictional boundaries were unclear and that instructions and general management of the incident were muddled. It is hoped that analysis of the confusion arising from this situation will lead ultimately to improved crisis management and a clearer definition of jurisdictional authority at all levels of government.

As mentioned previously, radioactivity released from TMI Unit 2 into the environment was composed principally of about 10 MCi of xenon-133 and 15 Ci of iodine-131. These nuclides produced an average radiation dose to the surrounding populace of about 8 mrem over a radius of 10 miles and about 2 mrem over a radius of 50 miles from TMI. From the most conservative estimates, these radiation doses might be expected to induce an additional 0.7 cancer deaths in the population of two million persons living within 50 miles of TMI.[4] The number of cancer deaths occurring spontaneously in this population is estimated at 330,000 over the lifetimes of the persons involved.

In all likelihood, the government and public response to the TMI incident will prove much more hazardous to the public health and safety than the incident itself. There is little question but that TMI has enhanced the burden on a nuclear power industry already weakened by public sentiment and government regulation and that the ultimate impact of the incident will be to increase the country's dependence on coal-fired electricity. As estimated by Sir Ernest Titterton,[6] this increased dependence will cause 100 additional mining and transportation deaths per year, as many as 125,000 cases per year of chronic respiratory disease, and perhaps 1 million person-days of aggravated heart-lung symptoms.

If the TMI incident has a lesson, it is that the United States needs a well-conceived and executed energy policy that reflects a thoughtful balance among all sources of energy production. Without such a policy, the United States undoubtedly will continue to struggle along without the sound energy foundation necessary for the economic stability and social security of an industrialized society.

REFERENCES

1. Martin D: *Three Mile Island.* Cambridge, Mass, Ballinger, 1980.
2. Stephens M: *Three Mile Island.* New York, Random House, 1980.
3. Rubinstein E: An analysis of Three Mile Island—The accident that shouldn't have happened. *IEEE Spectrum* 1979; 16 (11),: 30–42.
4. *The Accident At Three Mile Island.* Report of the President's Commission. US Government Printing Office, 1979.
5. Barker B (ed): Prelude: The accident at Three Mile Island. *Electric Power Res Inst* 1980; 7–13.
6. Titterton E: Risk, safety, costs and common sense. *Interdisciplinary Science Rev* 1981; 6 (4): 333–339.

Index

259